INSTANT WISDOM
FOR GPs

Every consultant has pearls of wisdom they wish they could share with GPs: knowledge they have acquired from years of experience and evidence-based study, which could lead to improved speed and decision in referral, more efficient use of resources and, overall, better patient care. *Instant Wisdom for GPs* gathers these pearls together, presenting ten bullet-point gems from a comprehensive range of clinical specialties, together with advice on obscure or overlooked diagnoses, guidance on how to distinguish tricky differentials and tips on prescribing.

The content has been thoroughly revised and updated for this second edition. New chapters have been added on alcohol use disorders, behavioural problems in children, clinical biochemistry, emergency presentations, genetics and genomics, obesity and bariatric medicine, and women's health, all from contributors expert in these fields.

Key features:

- Each specialty chapter offers ten pearls of wisdom, with detailed explanation from a leading consultant
- 'Obscure or overlooked diagnoses' flag conditions which the GP might not have heard about or might overlook or confuse with others
- 'Easily confused' sections highlight at-a-glance diagnoses which can be challenging to distinguish from each other, presented in an easy-to-read table
- 'Prescribing points' in each chapter highlight relevant issues around prescribing, including tips, warnings and clarifications
- Fully revised and updated with seven new chapters

Edited by **Keith Hopcroft**, author of the critically acclaimed *Symptom Sorter*, this practical and accessible guide distils years of knowledge, experience and key evidence into 32 concise and easy-to-navigate chapters and is essential reading for trainee and practising GPs.

INSTANT WISDOM
FOR GPs

PEARLS FROM ALL THE SPECIALTIES

Second Edition

EDITED BY **KEITH HOPCROFT**

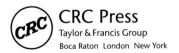

CRC Press
Taylor & Francis Group
Boca Raton   London   New York

CRC Press is an imprint of the
Taylor & Francis Group, an **informa** business

CONTENTS

PREFACE

I'm fairly confident that if anyone was dispensing instant wisdom on writing a book, they would say that no one ever reads a preface. On that basis, I'll keep this brief.

The idea for this project has been kicking around in my brain for years. Partly because I've always loved those wise nuggets you occasionally pick up from a particularly good lecture or article. And partly because of the event that spawned Pearl 20 in the 'General practice' chapter. Essentially, the book is an attempt to distil and collate gems of wisdom about medicine – derived from study, evidence, teaching and, especially, years of experience – that we all possess and might remember/reveal if we were held upside down and shaken long enough.

Of course, true wisdom can't be instilled by digesting a book. But something quite close perhaps can be, and it was an attractive enough notion for me to have a go.

The logical way to structure the book is by speciality. As it will be of most interest to generalists – trainees, young GPs and established old-timers like me who still genuinely learn something every day – I sincerely hope it comes across as true enlightenment rather than unrealistic specialist dogma. If it errs towards the latter, then I've failed in my editing duties. The fact that I've contrived the 'General practice' chapter to be twice as long as all the others is some sort of insurance policy for this, plus it reflects the fact that, of course, general practice is the most difficult and wide-ranging speciality of all.

As for how you read the book, that's up to you. Dip in and out, or plough through methodically, as the fancy takes you. But I do hope it is read – and that, as a result, you feel that bit wiser, and your patients feel that bit better.

ACKNOWLEDGEMENTS

Frankly, I've lost track of all the people I should thank, there have been so many. But special mentions to Richard Davenport, Nick Summerton, Shaba Nabi and Alistair Moulds. Hats off to CRC Press/Taylor & Francis for taking the idea, and me, seriously. Obviously, a massive thank you to all the authors for turning around such high-quality work within my deadline, with only a few needing the cattle-prod treatment (they know who they are). And, lastly, I'd like to thank and dedicate the book to all GPs and their staff – and especially those at Laindon Medical Group – because it's their wisdom and their hard work that keeps the NHS afloat.

EDITOR

Keith Hopcroft has been a GP for 35 years, and is an ex-trainer and currently a tutor for students from Anglia Ruskin University. He has also written books for the public and the profession (including *Symptom Sorter*) and regular articles and columns for almost every national newspaper, plus longstanding columns and blogs for the profession press. He is an editorial adviser for Pulse.

CONTRIBUTORS

Helen Ashby
Consultant in Chemical Pathology and
Metabolic Medicine
Royal Wolverhampton NHS Trust
Wolverhampton, United Kingdom

David S. Baldwin
Professor of Psychiatry
Section Head, Clinical Neurosciences
University of Southampton
Southampton, United Kingdom

Elizabeth Ball
Consultant Gynaecologist
Royal London Hospital Barts Health
and
Honorary Reader
City University London
London, United Kingdom

Andrew Bath
Consultant ENT Surgeon
Norfolk and Norwich University
Hospital
NHS Foundation Trust
Norwich, United Kingdom

Tak Chin
Consultant Allergist
University Hospital Southampton
Southampton, United Kingdom

Wei Meng Chin
Consultant Community Paediatrician
East and North Hertfordshire NHS
Trust
Stevenage, United Kingdom

Tahseen A. Chowdhury
Consultant Diabetologist
Barts Health NHS Trust
and
Department of Diabetes
Royal London Hospital
London, United Kingdom

Phil Clelland
Registrar
Sports and Exercise Medicine
NW Deanery, United Kingdom

Stephanie Cooper
Speech and Language Therapist
Norfolk and Norwich University
Hospital
NHS Foundation Trust
Norwich, United Kingdom

Richard Davenport
Consultant Neurologist
Royal Infirmary of Edinburgh
Edinburgh, United Kingdom
and

Honorary Senior Lecturer
University of Edinburgh
Edinburgh, United Kingdom

Ian Eardley
Consultant Urologist
Leeds Teaching Hospital Trust
Leeds, United Kingdom

Matthew Harries
Consultant Dermatologist
Salford Royal Hospital
Northern Care Alliance NHS Foundation
Trust
Salford, United Kingdom
and
Senior Lecturer
University of Manchester,
Manchester, United Kingdom

Dylan Harris
Consultant
Palliative Medicine
Cwm Taf Morgannwg University Health
Board
and
Lecturer
Cardiff University
Wales, United Kingdom

Jude Hayward
GP in Shipley
GPwSI Genetics
Yorkshire Regional Genetics Service
and
Honorary Research Fellow
St. George's University London
and
Primary Care Adviser to Health
Education England
Genomics Education Programme
and

RCGP Joint Clinical Champion
Genomics Medicine
London, United Kingdom

Toni Hazell
GP
Somerset Gardens Family Healthcare
Centre
and
Board Member
Primary Care Women's Health Forum
London, United Kingdom

Peter Heinz
Consultant
Acute and General Paediatrics
Addenbrooke's Hospital
Cambridge, United Kingdom

Andy Hughes
Former Consultant
Community Haematologist
Mid and South Essex NHS Foundation
Trust
Essex, United Kingdom

Tom Hughes
Consultant Nephrologist
Basildon and Thurrock University
Hospitals
Basildon, United Kingdom

Aroon Lal
Consultant Nephrologist
Basildon and Thurrock University
Hospitals
Basildon, United Kingdom
and
Honorary Associate Clinical Professor
UCL Medical School
University College London
London, United Kingdom

John Leach
Consultant Neurosurgeon
Manchester, United Kingdom

Dalia Ludwig
Rheumatology Consultant
University College London Hospitals
NHS Foundation Trust
London, United Kingdom

Jessica J. Manson
Rheumatology Consultant
University College London Hospitals
NHS Foundation Trust
London, United Kingdom

Jerome Ment
Consultant Cardiologist
University Hospitals Birmingham
NHS Foundation Trust
Birmingham, United Kingdom

Stephen J. Middleton
Honorary Consultant
Gastroenterologist
Cambridge University Hospitals
Cambridge, United Kingdom

John Phillips
Consultant ENT Surgeon
Norfolk and Norwich University
Hospital
NHS Foundation Trust
Norwich, United Kingdom

Imran Rafi
Reader Primary Care and Genomics
Institute for Medical and Biomedical
Education
St George's, University of London
and
RCGP Joint Clinical Champion in
Genomics Medicine
London, United Kingdom

Omar Rafiq
Consultant Ophthalmologist
Moorfields Eye Hospital
Abu Dhabi, UAE

Michael Rayment
Consultant
Sexual Health and HIV
Medicine,
Chelsea and Westminster NHS
Foundation Trust
and
Honorary Senior Clinical
Lecturer
Imperial College London
London, United Kingdom

N.F.W. Redwood
Consultant General and Vascular
Surgeon (retired)

Adam Rosenthal
Consultant Gynaecologist
University College London
Hospitals
NHS Foundation Trust
and
Honorary Associate Professor
University College London
London, United Kingdom

David Rutkowski
The Dermatology Centre
University of Manchester
Salford Royal Hospital
Northern Care Alliance NHS
Foundation Trust
Salford, United Kingdom
and
Withington Community
Hospital
Manchester Foundation Trust
Manchester, United Kingdom

Zak Shakanti
The Dermatology Centre
University of Manchester
Salford Royal Hospital
Northern Care Alliance NHS
Foundation Trust
Salford, United Kingdom

Lisa M. Sharkey
Consultant Gastroenterologist
Cambridge University Hospitals
Cambridge, United Kingdom

Karol Sikora
Medical Director
Cancer Partners International
and
Founding Dean
University of Buckingham Medical
School
and
Former Professor and Chairman
Department of Cancer Medicine
Imperial College School of Medicine
London, United Kingdom

Julia Sinclair
Professor
Addiction Psychiatry, Faculty of
Medicine
University of Southampton
and
Honorary Consultant in Alcohol Liaison
University Hospital Southampton
Southampton
and
National Specialty Adviser for Alcohol
Dependence
NHS England
London, United Kingdom

Minal Singh
The Dermatology Centre
University of Manchester
Salford Royal Hospital
Northern Care Alliance NHS
Foundation Trust
Salford, United Kingdom
and
Division of Medical Education
School of Medical Sciences
University of Manchester
Manchester, United Kingdom

Jay Suntharalingam
Consultant Respiratory Physician
Respiratory Department
Royal United Hospitals Bath NHS
Foundation Trust
and
Visiting Professor
University of Bath
Bath, United Kingdom

Peter Tassone
Consultant ENT Surgeon
Norfolk and Norwich University
Hospital
NHS Foundation Trust
Norwich, United Kingdom

Mark P.J. Vanderpump
Consultant Physician and
Endocrinologist
OneWelbeck Endocrinology
London, United Kingdom

Charlotte Wing
Rheumatology Consultant
West Hertfordshire Teaching Hospitals
NHS Trust
Hertfordshire, United Kingdom

James Woodard
Consultant Geriatrician
Derby Teaching Hospitals NHS
Foundation Trust
Derby, United Kingdom

ALCOHOL USE DISORDERS

Julia Sinclair

Ten Pearls of Wisdom

1. ### Know your numbers; be able to estimate a (ballpark) figure of how much people drink

   One unit of alcohol in the UK is 10 mL (or 8 g) of pure ethanol. What does this mean in practice? A drink that is 40% alcohol by volume (ABV) has 40 units in 1 L, 20 units in 0.5 L and 10 units in 0.25 L, which means 1 unit is 25 mL (which is what you would be served in a bar as a 'single' shot). There is no need for mental arithmetic – going through it using pencil and paper with a patient is in itself a brief intervention (see Pearl 4). Many patients (especially if they are drinking at dependent levels) will be able to tell you the ABV % of what they drink, as they are often looking to maximise alcohol strength by price. Even with limited personal knowledge of alcohol-containing beverages, every clinician should be able to gain a good estimate of alcohol consumption by asking about the approximate strength, volume and frequency of alcohol consumed.

2. ### Never use 'CAGE' again

   The four questions that constitute the CAGE mnemonic (cut down, annoyed, guilty, eye-opener) give no objective assessment of the frequency and quantity of alcohol use. It has low sensitivity for identifying non-dependent levels of alcohol consumption, which may still be significant contributors to the patient's mental state or physical health. In addition, it goes against all the principles of motivational interviewing to encourage behaviour change and is likely to be countertherapeutic. The World Health Organization's recommended screening tool is the Alcohol Use Disorder Identification Test (AUDIT), and the first three (consumption) questions (AUDIT-C) are well validated for use in primary care.

3. ### Think of alcohol consumption on a spectrum

   In the same way that monitoring a patient's blood pressure, cholesterol level, weight and smoking habits facilitate a discussion around levels of risk and

DOI: 10.1201/9781003304586-1

potential interventions, so too does asking approximately how much someone is drinking and how often. Self-report is the only cost-effective solution for doing this in clinical practice, and the evidence is that patients expect to be asked. Ascertaining from everyone how far above (or below) the 'lower risk level' of 14 units of alcohol/per week they are reduces any defensiveness people feel about being asked. Over 80% of the population drink alcohol, and they are seeing you because they have a health concern – so it is relevant to ask.

4. Screening and brief intervention (SBI), or identification and brief advice (IBA), is less complex than it sounds

SBI and IBA are interchangeable terms for asking a patient about their alcohol consumption (see Pearl 1) and then reflecting with them about where their consumption is on the risk scale (above or below 14 units/week) – and, if necessary, giving them a leaflet or link to one of the many helpful websites with further information. The evidence is substantial that this simple 'clinical conversation' has a number needed to treat (NNT) of about eight in terms of significant reduction by a whole risk level in drinking (i.e. from increased to lower-risk drinking).

5. Drink diaries are the most effective (and empowering) tool for behaviour change

I love drink diaries – and keep one myself! They can be an essential part of 'watchful waiting' for patients with depression and anxiety, or before prescribing a proton pump inhibitor (PPI), antihypertensive, night sedation or any of the myriad things people present with that are maintained by alcohol consumed at increased risk levels (>14 units/week). Keeping a prospective log of alcohol consumption is frequently eye-opening for people and empowers them to make changes or maintain good habits. The key thing is to encourage people to see them as a tool to give direct feedback about their alcohol use; it is not to 'prove' to the clinician that they don't drink much. Encouraging patients to keep one assiduously for a couple of weeks is to primarily inform themselves (not you) about their consumption. Asking people about their progress and congratulating them on small positive changes is an effective intervention.

6. Red wine is not good for you

Unless, that is, you are a postmenopausal woman who drinks fewer than 5 units (two medium glasses of 13.5% red wine) per week. For everyone else, the 'beneficial' antioxidants and polyphenols can be found elsewhere, without the risks from alcohol. The drinks industry has done a good job in selling 'moderate' and 'responsible' levels of drinking, minimising the risks and expanding any 'positive' effect of alcohol well beyond the data.

7. Mind your language

For someone who is well integrated into Alcoholics Anonymous (AA), their self-identification as 'an alcoholic' is often a helpful part of their identity and determination to remain abstinent. For most other people, drinking at either increased risk or dependent levels the fear of being labelled 'an alcoholic' may prevent them from feeling able to discuss their level of alcohol consumption with you. Alcohol 'misuse' and 'abuse' are also unhelpful terms that understandably make people feel defensive. Many people who drink dependently feel a great deal of shame about their alcohol consumption, and others fear it will result in them being deprived of healthcare. The new US diagnostic classification of alcohol use disorders (mild, moderate, severe) is a useful development that recognises the spectrum of alcohol consumption and alcohol harms. Other helpful terms include 'alcohol dependence', 'alcohol-related harm' (e.g. liver disease) and being 'alcohol-free'.

8. Addiction is a form of enslavement

Part of the syndrome of alcohol dependence (or severe alcohol use disorder) is that an individual loses control and continues to drink despite evidence of harm to themselves or others (physical, mental or social). This loss of control engenders significant shame and self-loathing in many individuals. Most people do not wish to be bad parents, partners or work colleagues, and the fact that they are unable to prioritise these relationships over drinking alcohol makes many feel hopeless and worthless. Like other biological drives, the need to drink when your body and mind have become dependent on alcohol is all powerful, but often not recognised at a conscious level; people simply cannot imagine how life without alcohol might be possible. Validating the challenges and suggesting small steps that may facilitate regaining control (see Pearl 5) is likely to be more helpful than telling people they shouldn't drink – they know! On average, in England, only 13% of people with alcohol dependence (AD) find their way to specialist services. Most people with AD will change their behaviour in response to salient events, tipping points and helpful conversations – potentially ones they have with their GP, even if you are not aware of the impact it has.

9. Do not start a detox without a plan for how to remain alcohol-free afterwards

Safely reducing alcohol from a high level of daily consumption to which the body has become tolerant is a necessary step. However, it is hard to predict the severity of alcohol withdrawal at different levels of alcohol consumption in different people. At very high levels (30-plus units of alcohol/day) this ideally needs to be undertaken in a specialist unit given the risks of withdrawal seizures and other complications (e.g. delirium tremens and Wernicke–Korsakoff syndrome). For people drinking at lower daily levels (<20 units a day), this can be done in the community with support and monitoring. A rule of thumb that can be offered for people insisting on cutting down from high levels without additional help would be a 10% drop in alcohol units every 3–4 days, but titrating against withdrawal symptoms (shakes/sweats), though this is not recommended for anyone who had a previous withdrawal seizure. It is often helpful to swap to alcohol in smaller 'packages' for people who have no control once a bottle is open. For example, 1 bottle of 12% wine (9 units) to 4 × 400 mL cans of 5.5% beer/cider (8.8 units). This can then be cut down by a can every 2–3 days. However it is achieved, the absolute essential is not to start the process until there is a clear plan for remaining alcohol-free once the 'detox' has finished. There is rarely any need to start an 'emergency' detox in the community, despite the pleadings of family members or the patient. The advice would be to monitor what they are drinking (see Pearl 5) while they engage with local community services or other agencies, and a longer-term plan for remaining alcohol-free can be made. Every time someone starts a detox and returns to drinking almost immediately is detrimental to their cognition and sense of self-efficacy, so reducing the likelihood of ultimately reaching a healthy stable recovery.

10. Stable recovery may take up to 5 years

For many people, especially those within the AA fellowship, 'recovery' is a lifelong process. For others, recovery happens at a point in time beyond which they no longer see their non-drinking status as anything other than a positive lifestyle choice that they are unlikely to change. As with all changes in behaviour, lapses happen and are best dealt with by expecting them and encouraging what can be learned from them.

Obscure and Overlooked Diagnoses

1. Wernicke–Korsakoff syndrome (WKS)

This is a form of alcohol-related brain injury. The acute presentation is rarely seen in primary care, as it is a complication of severe alcohol withdrawal and requires immediate hospital admission and treatment with parenteral thiamine. However, many patients gradually develop the executive dysfunction and memory problems of WKS, masked by ongoing alcohol consumption. It is characterised by impairment of retrieval of recent memories and results in 'confabulation' where in response to a question (e.g. 'What did you have for breakfast?') a categorical answer will be given (e.g. 'a piece of toast') in the absence of being able to retrieve the memory of what they actually ate. With a collateral history, this is quickly clear. Other than working with the family to put a plan in place to reduce and stop drinking (see Pearl 9), advising a good diet and prescribing thiamine (see later), there is sadly very little currently available for these patients.

2. **'Holiday heart syndrome'**

   This is an alcohol-induced atrial arrhythmia presenting after a period (a week or long weekend) of excessive alcohol consumption, stress or dehydration in an otherwise healthy person without other clinical evidence of heart disease. A good history and exclusion of other underlying causes are key to management. If otherwise clinically stable, management is reassurance; advise about alcohol cessation and consideration of the risk for also developing other health conditions (see next).

3. **Alcohol as a causative/contributory factor in various pathologies**

   Elevated alcohol consumption is frequently a predisposing, precipitating or maintaining cause or contributory factor for:

   - Depression
   - Generalised anxiety disorder
   - Panic attacks
   - High blood pressure
   - Gastritis
   - Pancreatitis
   - Insomnia
   - Sexual dysfunction
   - Menopausal symptoms
   - Obesity
   - Peripheral neuropathy
   - Inflammatory conditions
   - Memory problems in older adults

Ask all patients with any long-term condition about their alcohol consumption as part of the range of self-management techniques. Alcohol consumption has a particularly complex interaction with chronic pain, which is frequently challenging to break but essential to acknowledge if any progress is to be made.

Easily Confused

1. **Alcohol-related or '-unrelated' morbidity**

   Alcohol is a small molecule, gets into every organ of the body, and is a poison (albeit a favourite one) – and so is a potential predisposing, precipitating or maintaining cause of many conditions. The following may all present as indistinguishable from the non-comorbid (with alcohol) disorder.

Presentation	Specific points for alcohol-related aspects	For all patients
Cognitive impairment	■ The only reversible form of dementia – a useful motivating technique	■ Ask about alcohol consumption as part of the range of self-management techniques
Depression	■ Manage concurrently ■ Antidepressants have some benefit if moderate/severe symptoms ■ Mirtazapine helpful with sleep ■ Risk of overdose increased	■ Encourage drink diaries (see Pearl 5)
Anxiety symptoms	■ Early symptom of alcohol withdrawal ■ Often consistently occurs at the end of workday – always settled by first drink	■ Reinforce that whatever the primary presentation, a reduction in alcohol consumption will improve symptoms
Insomnia	■ May get worse for a week or two after stopping drinking ■ Prepare people for this and encourage sleep hygiene ■ In the recently abstinent, check they are not replacing alcohol with caffeine/ energy drinks	
Sexual dysfunction	■ Very quickly reversible – a useful motivating technique	■ Active management of both conditions is more effective than getting into futile 'chicken and egg' debates
Menopausal symptoms	■ Reduction/cessation of alcohol may significantly improve symptoms	
Obesity	■ Alcohol is a high-calorie, nutrient-poor foodstuff ■ Simpler to cut out alcohol than other food swaps	
Peripheral neuropathy	■ In heavy drinkers, needs active management ■ Prescribe thiamine and other B vitamins	
High blood pressure	■ Dose-dependent relationship of consumption with blood pressure ■ In recently abstinent, review need for antihypertensives	

2. Alcohol-related liver disease (ARLD)

There is confusion about who should be tested and how.

■ Alcohol-related liver disease (ARLD) develops silently for 10–15 years.

■ Consider ARLD in men drinking >50 units/week and women drinking >35 units/week who have been doing so for some months.

■ Follow local liver pathway for screening (refer for FibroScan/ELF test, etc., which can identify and stage liver disease).

■ Standard liver function tests (alkaline phosphatase [ALP], alanine transaminase [ALT]) are not useful for screening for ARLD.

■ Over 50% of people with alcohol dependence have normal ALP/ALT.

■ Refer to hepatology if ALT is up, plus there are signs of chronic liver disease.

Prescribing Points

1. **Thiamine (and other B vitamins) can be lifesaving**
   They are essential in the metabolism of carbohydrates (including alcohol), so people who are drinking daily, have high levels of requirement and have poor nutritional intake and absorption are likely to be deficient. Oral replacement may be a useful form of harm minimisation until alcohol-free and eating properly (1 to 2 months after becoming abstinent). However, given the poor oral absorption, if the patient is at imminent risk of WKS, parenteral thiamine replacement is required (see 'Obscure and overlooked diagnoses').

2. **Relapse prevention medications do work**
   They have an NNT of between 8 and 12 and are usually most effective when combined with psychosocial interventions, though that may be support from family or friends. Not being able to engage with local treatment services is not a reason not to prescribe if people are otherwise committed to abstinence. NICE recommendations are that they are prescribed for 6 to 12 months.
   - *Acamprosate*: Start early to help with the tail end of withdrawal symptoms. It is safe and well tolerated, with no abuse liability. For some, the act of taking tablets three times a day is a helpful regular reminder of their intention to remain abstinent. For those unwilling to take six tablets daily, there is not much point in starting it, as the dose will likely be subtherapeutic. Stop if the patient returns to daily drinking – it is most effective for the maintenance of abstinence, rather than preventing a return to heavy drinking.
   - *Naltrexone*: An opioid antagonist, and so works indirectly by reducing craving and limiting the reinforcing effects of alcohol if someone lapses, preventing a full-blown relapse. It is less well tolerated than acamprosate (particularly in women), but only requires one tablet a day, which may help some with adherence. The main limitation of prescribing is blocking the effect of any opioid – so it is contraindicated in patients prescribed opioids. It is most effective at preventing a return to heavy drinking, rather than maintenance of abstinence, and patients should be encouraged to stay on it if they have a lapse.
   - *Disulfiram (Antabuse)*: This blocks the enzyme aldehyde dehydrogenase, so alcohol is metabolised to toxic acetaldehyde. It is still a very useful drug for some people who find the 'psychological threat' helpful and are willing to adhere to the alcohol-related dietary restrictions. For some patients, the absorption of alcohol in perfumes and mouthwash may also cause a reaction and need to be avoided. Always start under specialist supervision. Some people who find it beneficial may wish to continue for years, in which case an annual review of liver function is required, given a (low) potential for toxicity,

which needs to be balanced against the potential for ARLD if the patient returns to drinking.

- *Baclofen*: An off-label drug that may be useful in patients with severe ARLD for whom all other relapse prevention medications are contraindicated. It should be initiated and monitored by a specialist only.

3. **Don't start benzodiazepines in people with alcohol dependence**
   Unless, that is, there is a very specific short-term indication. It is likely to result in dependence on both substances and make reduction from both more complex.

ALLERGY

Tak Chin

Ten Pearls of Wisdom

1. **A high total IgE does not necessarily indicate allergic disease and a normal total IgE does not exclude allergy**

   Immunoglobulin E (IgE) is the antibody that mediates allergic reactions; however, measuring total IgE is not useful in the management of allergic diseases. Total IgE in the circulation includes IgE antibodies directed against allergens (allergen-specific IgE) and infective agents, plus some are of unknown specificity. Hence, total IgE can be high in the absence of allergic disease. On the other hand, a patient may have specific IgE against an allergen (e.g. cat), while the total IgE may not exceed the normal range. For allergy diagnosis, it is better to measure allergen-specific IgE against an allergen suspected from the history.

2. **'Chronic urticaria and/or angioedema' is usually non-allergic**

   Urticaria and angioedema are relatively common, although often transient, conditions. Urticaria is also known as hives or nettle rash, and angioedema appears as diffuse swelling. Acute urticaria and/or angioedema (one-off episodes) could result from an allergic reaction (such as to foods or drugs) or from infection. However, some patients present with recurrent episodes of urticaria and/or angioedema not associated with any specific or consistent trigger (although note Pearl 7 regarding patients on ACE inhibitors). These patients are usually suffering from spontaneous (idiopathic) urticaria and/or angioedema, which is not due to allergy. Chronic spontaneous urticaria and/or angioedema involve skin and/or mucous membrane, and only rarely progresses to anaphylaxis. These patients require reassurance and treatment with (high-dose, if needed) antihistamines.

3. **Only a small proportion of adverse reactions to drugs are due to drug allergy**

   Adverse reactions to drugs can be expected (related to their pharmacological effects) and unexpected. For pharmacological adverse effects, consider dose adjustment or use of an alternative medication. The 'unexpected' reactions could be due to allergy, intolerance or idiosyncrasy. An allergic reaction has

DOI: 10.1201/9781003304586-2

9

an immunological basis, although that may not be easy to establish. Hence, for practical purposes, any drug reaction with clinical features of allergy (such as rash or anaphylaxis) can be regarded as allergic. There is usually no simple test to diagnose drug allergy, and drug provocation tests are often required to establish the diagnosis. These are cumbersome and carry significant risks. Therefore, if possible, consideration should be given to using a suitable alternative before referral for drug allergy testing. If no suitable alternative is available, however, patients should be referred for testing and if drug allergy is confirmed, desensitisation is possible, which would allow safe use of the drug.

4. Avoid indiscriminate penicillin prescribing in children if possible – the child may end up with a lifelong erroneous label of penicillin allergy

Penicillin and its derivatives belong to the beta-lactam group of antibiotics that share a beta-lactam ring structure, which also includes cephalosporins. Approximately 10% of the population reports an allergy to penicillin, but only 1% are confirmed following formal testing. Many of these patients were given a penicillin group of antibiotics during childhood for a viral illness with the viral exanthem wrongly labelled as penicillin allergic rash. They are subsequently advised to avoid penicillins, resulting in more costly and less safe alternative antibiotics given throughout their life unnecessarily. This emphasises the need to try to avoid antibiotic prescribing in childhood viral illnesses.

5. All patients with an anaphylaxis of unknown cause should be referred to an allergy clinic

Most anaphylaxis guidelines recommend that all patients with a new or unexpected anaphylactic episode should be referred to an allergy specialist to investigate possible triggers in order to minimise the risk of future reactions and to provide a management plan. This is done with a detailed history, allergy skin prick, and/or intradermal testing, blood tests and, if required, provocation tests to identify the allergic cause and institute preventive measures. If food is involved, referral to a specialist dietitian is helpful. Contact information for patient support groups (such as Anaphylaxis UK) may be helpful.

6. Pollen-food allergy syndrome/oral allergy syndrome is often unrecognised or misdiagnosed

This is an increasingly common phenomenon seen in adults with hay fever. It is caused by cross-reacting proteins found in pollen, which are similar to proteins found in raw fruits, vegetables or tree nuts. As a result, the body mistakes the food proteins for pollen proteins and so the immune system reacts to them.

The foods most likely to cause pollen-food allergy syndrome in birch pollen allergy (the most common form) are raw apple, kiwi fruit, peach, cherry, other stone fruits, hazelnut and almond. The reactions are usually limited to oral itching, tingling or swelling only (hence it is also called oral allergy syndrome), which occurs within minutes of eating the cross-reactive foods. There is usually no systemic involvement or cardiovascular compromise. Another typical feature of pollen-food allergy syndrome is that patients are usually able to tolerate the cooked, processed or tinned forms of the raw foods which cause problems (as heating and processing breaks down the causative proteins).

7. **Consider ACE-induced angioedema in those taking the relevant drug who suffer from intermittent oral angioedema – even if they have been on the treatment for years**

   Check medication lists for ACE inhibitors in patients presenting with angioedema that only affects the lips, tongue or face. There is no associated urticaria or other features of anaphylaxis.

   The mechanism of ACE-induced angioedema is not allergic. While it is an easy diagnosis to pick up when ACE inhibitors have just been started, ACE-induced angioedema more often occurs after many years of uneventful use. As a result, many patients have recurrent episodes of orofacial angioedema before the diagnosis is made.

8. **Consider referral of certain patients with wasp or bee sting anaphylaxis for insect venom immunotherapy (which is available on the NHS)**

   Patients who have anaphylaxis to wasp or bee stings can be desensitised with venom immunotherapy, which is usually given as a 3-year course of injections. This is a very effective treatment and is successful in preventing systemic reactions in approximately 95%–100% of wasp venom allergy patients and approximately 80% of bee venom allergy patients. Those at high risk of future stings (such as gardeners or beekeepers) should be considered for venom immunotherapy.

9. **Eczema in adulthood is rarely due to food allergy**

   While studies have shown that certain foods such as cow's milk and egg can exacerbate eczema in more than 50% of children of preschool age, similar reactions to 'classical' food allergens are not common in adults. Food allergy should certainly be considered in infants with severe eczema. An allergy skin prick test and/or oral food challenge may help to identify the cause; however, finding a 'causative' food for eczema in adulthood is very rare. Unnecessary dietary restrictions that are not based on proper diagnosis may lead to malnutrition and additional psychological stress.

10. **Skin prick testing and patch testing are very different – know which to use and when**

    These are very different tests. Skin prick testing is helpful for type I IgE-mediated allergic reactions (e.g. foods and aeroallergens), whereas patch testing is helpful for type IV delayed-type hypersensitivity reactions (e.g. fragrances, chemicals and metals). Skin prick testing can be performed in 15 minutes, while patch testing is usually done over the course of 5 days (patches applied on day 1 with further appointments on days 3 and 5 to read the results). Patch testing is usually done to investigate contact allergies by dermatologists rather than allergists.

Obscure or Overlooked Diagnoses

1. **Food-dependent exercise-induced anaphylaxis**
   Exercise is a known physical factor that can trigger anaphylaxis. In some patients, food can act as a cofactor – this is known as 'food-dependent exercise-induced anaphylaxis'. Food can be ingested safely by itself, but the association with exercise is crucial for the onset of symptoms. This is seen more often in adults than in children. The most common food implicated is wheat. The most frequently reported exercise associated with food-dependent exercise-induced anaphylaxis is jogging/running. A provocation test is required if there is doubt regarding the diagnosis. Management includes avoidance of eating the suspected food 4 hours before exercise and carrying an adrenaline auto-injector.

2. **Baboon syndrome (symmetrical drug-related intertriginous and flexural exanthema [SDRIFE])**
   This is a reaction that results in a distinctive erythematous rash affecting the skin folds. When it predominantly affects the buttocks and natal cleft, it resembles the red bottom of a baboon (hence its name). The neck, armpits, flexures and other skin folds may also be affected symmetrically. It is usually caused by systemic exposure to drugs (such as beta-lactam antibiotics).

3. **Aquagenic urticaria**
   This is not technically an allergy to water, but rather a very rare form of physical urticaria (now classified as inducible urticaria), where hives develop immediately on contact with water regardless of temperature. It is not IgE-mediated.
   It typically presents in early teenagers and tends to affect young women. Reactions tend to occur with activities such as bathing, swimming or walking in the rain.

4. **Seminal plasma allergy**
   This is a rare condition affecting women that causes allergic reactions to semen. It is caused by developing a specific IgE antibody response to proteins in seminal fluid (rather than the spermatozoa). Reactions usually occur after unprotected intercourse and vary from localised pain to generalised systemic reactions (including anaphylaxis).

Easily Confused

1. Allergic urticaria and spontaneous/idiopathic urticaria

Allergic urticaria	Spontaneous/idiopathic urticaria
■ Consistent trigger ■ Immediate reaction within 5–15 minutes of exposure to trigger ■ Present only on exposure to allergen	■ No consistent trigger ■ No consistent timing with reaction to suspected trigger ■ If present most days for more than 6 weeks, then an allergen is unlikely

2. Food allergy and food intolerance/irritable bowel syndrome

Food allergy	Food intolerance/irritable bowel syndrome
■ Is immunologically mediated ■ Reactions are acute (within minutes of ingestion) ■ Multisystem manifestation (skin, gastrointestinal, respiratory, cardiovascular) ■ Could be fatal ■ Is more common in children ■ Common suspected foods are milk, egg, nuts, seafood and fruits ■ Strict avoidance is required	■ Food can be a non-immunological trigger ■ Reactions can be delayed after ingestion of suspected food ■ Clinical manifestations are generally confined to gastrointestinal tract ■ Not fatal ■ Is more common in adults ■ Common suspected foods are grains ■ Avoidance need not be strict

Prescribing Points

1. High-dose antihistamines are generally safe

Non-sedating antihistamines are the mainstay of treatment for chronic urticaria, and up to four times the recommended dose can be used. However, at high doses, many non-sedating antihistamines can manifest sedating properties. Fexofenadine is better tolerated in terms of sedating effects even at higher doses. Antihistamines should be avoided in pregnancy if possible; however, no teratogenic effects have been reported, and there is considerable clinical experience of safety with cetirizine and loratadine during pregnancy.

2. Start hay fever medications about 1 month before the start of the pollen season

Hay fever medications are most effective if they are started a few weeks before pollen is released. Starting hay fever medications in this way (as opposed to when allergy symptoms have developed and allergic inflammation has already become established) reduces or even prevents the release of histamine and other allergic mediators, which results in less severe symptoms. Trees typically release pollen from March to May; with grasses, typically, the key time is May to August.

3. **Beware that ARBs can cause angioedema too**

   In patients who have had ACE-induced angioedema who need to be switched to a different class of antihypertensive, be aware that there is a risk of developing angioedema with angiotensin II receptor blockers (ARBs) (risk reported to be 0%–9.2% to 2%–17%). If after risk assessment it is felt that an ARB is clinically required, this should be discussed with the patient and they should be adequately counselled.

4. **Treatment of anaphylaxis is with intramuscular adrenaline**

   Anaphylaxis, defined as a systemic, life-threatening allergic reaction, should be treated immediately with intramuscular administration of adrenaline (conveniently available as adrenaline auto-injector devices). For adults and older children, the usual dose is 0.30 to 0.50 mg. For paediatric use, the usual dose is 0.15 to 0.30 mg depending upon the body weight of the patient (approximate guide 0.01 mg/kg body weight). Intravenous or intramuscular antihistamines and corticosteroids are additional secondary treatments. High-flow oxygen and inhaled or nebulised bronchodilators may be administered if there is evidence of bronchoconstriction. Once stable, patients should be transferred to the hospital as delayed reactions do occasionally occur.

Acknowledgements to S. Hasan Arshad and Elizabeth Griffiths for previous contributions in first edition.

CARDIOLOGY

Jerome Ment

Ten Pearls of Wisdom

1. **The key factor with anginal pain is the consistent relation to exertion and an easing with rest**

   Ischaemic symptoms may have many modes of presentation, often specific to an individual patient. Typical angina is often described as a central chest heaviness or tightness with exertion, but cardiac ischaemia can manifest as pain from anywhere from the jaw to the umbilicus, or even the back. The most important feature is the clear relationship with exercise – and the fact that it usually remains consistent in nature for an individual patient.

2. **Beware that patients may have more than one type of chest pain**

   It is not unusual for a patient to describe atypical chest pain, often easily explained as musculoskeletal, which can mask the more typical manifestations of angina unless these are carefully elicited. So, in patients with appropriate risk factors, ask about exertional symptoms and changes in exercise capacity, even if the history is initially suggestive of musculoskeletal pain. Conversely, patients with known ischaemic heart disease may experience non-cardiac chest pain. After a myocardial infarction, patients often become very aware of their heart and chest and may describe 'twinges' of short-lived, localised, often left-sided chest pain unrelated to activity. Early reassurance can be invaluable in settling these symptoms before they escalate and raise concerns.

3. **Cardiac ischaemia may manifest as breathlessness rather than pain**

   Some patients with cardiac ischaemia will report breathlessness as the sole symptom. While this is most often described in patients with diabetes, it can occur in non-diabetics too. The breathlessness is exertional, particularly on inclines or stairs, and eases quickly with rest and is often worse in cold weather. Typically, there is an absence of accompanying respiratory symptoms such as a productive cough or wheeze. On more detailed enquiry, patients will sometimes describe short-lived chest tightness with exercise, but the dominant symptom is the sensation of breathlessness.

DOI: 10.1201/9781003304586-3

4. Don't be misled by the 'walk through' phenomenon

Some patients with angina experience a 'warm up' or 'walk through' phenomenon which can confuse the unwary clinician. These patients begin to experience their typical angina on exertion, but over time some discover that if they can continue for a little longer, their symptoms dissipate, allowing them to 'walk through' the symptom. This phenomenon, usually ascribed to ischaemic preconditioning – an adaptive response whereby repeated short periods of ischaemia protect the heart against a subsequent ischaemic insult – is considered protective to some degree but needs to be recognised as part of the spectrum of angina symptoms.

5. Automated ECG interpretation is not always correct

Modern ECG machines can provide automated interpretation to aid the clinician. Unfortunately, this can be misleading and often plain wrong, raising anxiety in both patient and doctor. The most common example is the 'consider previous inferior infarct' report; in fact, T wave inversion and small Q waves in one or two inferior leads are often normal. Other common examples include movement artefact interpreted as atrial fibrillation, and QT interval prolongation where the U wave and not the T wave has been measured. It is worth double checking, or getting a cardiologist to review the ECG, if the automated interpretation is out of step with the clinical picture.

6. Significant palpitations are usually sustained, exertional and/or accompanied by other symptoms

The symptom of palpitations is one of the most common reasons for referral to cardiology, yet in many cases, patients can be reassured that their symptoms are harmless. They will typically describe short-lived flutters, often at rest or in bed at night, accompanied by 'missed beats' typical of benign isolated ectopic beats. More significant symptoms are suggested by sustained palpitations with a 'heart racing' phenomenon, particularly if exertional and accompanied by dizziness or chest pain. Ask about a family history of sudden cardiac death or premature heart attacks. If present, this warrants early referral and investigation.

7. Heart failure is very difficult to diagnose clinically

Systolic heart failure is an important and life-limiting diagnosis that can now be effectively treated, if not cured; however, clinical diagnosis can be fraught with difficulty. In one study, cardiologists were only able to correctly diagnose it at the bedside in 40% of cases. Ankle swelling, breathlessness and lung crepitations are poor discriminators. More specific markers are a displaced apex beat, a raised venous pressure and the presence of a systolic murmur at the apex. BNP, while often used as a screening tool, lacks specificity and a raised BNP in isolation should not be regarded as confirmation of the diagnosis. An abnormal ECG, particularly in the presence of a left bundle branch block or atrial fibrillation, should raise the level of suspicion further. An echocardiogram remains the gold standard test and may also offer insights into the underlying aetiology.

8. Cardiac symptoms aren't always caused by coronary atheroma

A number of cardiac conditions can present with one or more of the three cardinal cardiac symptoms: chest pain, breathlessness and syncope. The elderly patient, in particular, should be examined carefully for aortic stenosis. The typical murmur requires prompt referral and investigation. Delays, or inappropriate investigation or treatment – such as exercise testing or sublingual nitrates – can have potentially fatal outcomes. In the younger patient, take a family history and ask about sudden cardiac death or cardiomyopathies. An ECG revealing left ventricular hypertrophy or widespread T wave inversion should also alert the clinician to an underlying and important cardiomyopathy.

9. Know the possible reasons for resistant hypertension – and consider spironolactone

Resistant hypertension can be extremely challenging. Addressing non-pharmacological factors may help. Obesity and high salt intake are recognised as contributors, but less well-known are the effects of alcohol and dietary indiscretions such as liquorice and excess caffeine. Obstructive sleep apnoea is another important association, effective treatment of which may significantly improve blood pressure control. Careful clinical enquiry of the patient, or more often the partner, will often help select patients for further investigative screening. Drug therapy is often more effective and better tolerated if used in combination and at mid-range doses, although compliance should always be confirmed before any adjustments. An underlying cause remains uncommon but should be sought in younger patients (under 40 years old), in drug-resistant hypertension despite three agents, or where clinical findings or baseline blood tests are suggestive. If all else fails, consider the addition of spironolactone, particularly in those with associated obesity where hyperaldosteronism may be more common.

10. Remember that hyperlipidaemia may have an underlying cause

Lipid profiles are one of the most commonly requested blood tests from general practice. Before reaching for the prescription pad, consider some important possible underlying causes. These include lifestyle factors such as excessive alcohol intake (raised triglycerides); a diet rich in saturated fats (total cholesterol, TG), particularly the now trendy Keto diet; a sedentary lifestyle and cigarette smoking (low HDL); as well as a number of systemic illnesses including hypothyroidism, diabetes mellitus, primary biliary cirrhosis and nephrotic syndrome. Finally, drugs such as antiretroviral agents, retinoids, cyclosporin and corticosteroids may also result in adverse lipid profiles.

Obscure or Overlooked Diagnoses

1. **Infective endocarditis**

   This usually involves cardiac valves but may affect other areas such as pacemaker leads. It is rare but potentially life-threatening. Patients may present with non-specific symptoms such as anorexia, weight loss, joint pain, fever and sweats. The chronic nature of these symptoms (weeks) should ring alarm bells. Clinically, a new murmur is the cardinal sign along with splinter haemorrhages. Investigations reveal microscopic haematuria and a raised white blood count and C-reactive protein. While it can affect anyone, patients most at risk are those with prosthetic valves, those on dialysis, intravenous drug users and patients with known congenital heart disease.

2. **Ischaemia with normal coronary arteries (INOCA)**

   This comprises typical angina that presents with evidence of ischaemia (30% of patients have abnormal myocardial perfusion scans) but with normal epicardial vessels. It is poorly understood, but putative mechanisms include microvascular dysfunction, coronary spasm and abnormal pain gating mechanisms. There is no universally accepted treatment; regimes are often established by trial and error. Treating additional risk factors may help, but the prognosis is good with low rates of severe adverse cardiac events.

3. **Takotsubo cardiomyopathy**

   Takotsubo cardiomyopathy, or broken heart syndrome, is characterised by severe, typical cardiac-sounding chest pain indicative of acute myocardial infarction often accompanied by ECG changes – yet no vessel occlusion is seen on coronary angiogram. The condition is often precipitated by acute emotional stress. The mechanism is unclear; acute severe catecholamine surge, microvascular dysfunction and coronary spasm are possible explanations. Patients need early and prompt admission to support the left ventricle – yet curiously, in most instances, there is complete recovery.

4. **Long QT syndrome**

   This is a genetic disorder resulting in the prolongation of the corrected QT interval with a resultant increased risk of ventricular arrhythmias or sudden cardiac death. There is usually nothing to find on clinical examination. The diagnosis needs to be considered in any patient presenting with syncope, particularly if there is a family history of sudden cardiac death. Patients need urgent referral to specialist cardiac and genetic clinics. Beta-blocker therapy is the mainstay of therapy and should be initiated as soon as the diagnosis is suspected or confirmed. More specialist treatment includes pacemaker or defibrillator implantation. More commonly seen is a prolonged QT interval sometimes associated with medications or electrolyte disorders such as hypokalaemia or hypomagnesaemia. While there is a multitude of drugs that may be associated with QT prolongation, some of the most common are antipsychotics such as quetiapine, antidepressants such as amitriptyline, and antibiotics and antifungals (erythromycin, levofloxacin and ketoconazole). The risk becomes most significant only once the corrected QT interval extends beyond 500 ms.

5. **Postural orthostatic tachycardia syndrome (POTS)**

Orthostatic tachycardia is defined as a rise in heart rate of more than 30 beats per minute or a sinus tachycardia (>120 beats/minute) within 10 minutes of standing. It is increasingly recognised as a form of dysautonomia and may present with various non-specific symptoms including fatigue, exercise intolerance, headache (orthostatic migraine), palpitations, lightheadedness or even syncope. Most patients are young women and symptoms may be severe. Formal diagnostic confirmation involves tilt testing, but a simple pulse check on standing is often enough to confirm orthostatic tachycardia. Other causes for dysautonomia – particularly diabetes – need to be ruled out. Patients should increase their fluid intake to 2 or 3 litres a day along with increased salt in the diet. Drug therapy includes fludrocortisone; beta-blockers or ivabradine, which is sometimes better tolerated; SSRIs; and midodrine, where postural hypotension is a dominant feature.

Easily Confused

1. **Supraventricular tachycardia (SVT) and anxiety**

	SVT	Overlapping symptoms/ findings	Anxiety
History	■ Predominant symptoms are an abrupt onset of palpitations with an awareness of a very rapid heartbeat followed sometimes by anxiety	■ Palpitations	■ Predominant symptom is anxiety, often with hyperventilation and a feeling of panic; an awareness of heartbeat may develop but does not trigger the other symptoms
Examination	■ Usually normal unless examined during SVT ■ During SVT, heart rate is usually over 150 beats/minute	■ Tachycardia	■ Usually normal unless during an episode ■ Tachycardia may be present but heart rates are usually well below 150 beats/minute ■ Other features include hyperventilation, anxiety and distress

(Continued)

Investigations	■ ECG confirms SVT if taken during an episode ■ May be terminated with vagal manoeuvres such as forced Valsalva/carotid sinus massage ■ Cardiac monitoring during symptoms demonstrates sudden onset rapid tachycardia/SVT		■ ECG shows normal/sinus tachycardia during episode ■ Vagal manoeuvres have no effect ■ Cardiac monitoring during symptoms demonstrates normal sinus rhythm/sinus tachycardia

2. Angina versus musculoskeletal pain

	Angina	*Overlapping symptoms/ findings*	*Musculoskeletal chest pain*
History	■ Pain diffuse ■ Dull ache/tightness ■ Comes on with exertion and eases with rest ■ Improves with sublingual nitrates	■ Chest pain	■ Pain localised ■ Sharp/stabbing pain ■ Often felt at rest and may be persistent, sometimes for hours or days ■ Improves with analgesia
Examination	■ Usually normal. An underlying cause can sometimes be found, e.g. aortic stenosis		■ Localised tenderness of the chest wall reproducing the pain ■ Neck tenderness with referred pain to the chest
Investigations	■ ECG – normal in 50% of patients with angina ■ Possible evidence of previous infarction ■ Ischaemic stress testing		■ ECG – usually normal ■ Stress testing – normal

3. Congestive cardiac failure (CCF) and chronic obstructive pulmonary disease (COPD)

	CCF	*Overlapping symptoms/ findings*	*COPD*
History	■ Cough if present is usually non-productive ■ Peripheral oedema common ■ Seen in non-smokers	■ Breathlessness ■ Cough	■ Symptoms predominated by productive cough ■ Peripheral oedema if present is often dependent ■ Rarely seen in lifelong non-smokers

(Continued)

Examination	■ Pitting oedema ■ Elevated JVP ■ Systolic murmurs (often mitral regurgitation) may be present ■ Fine basal crepitations ■ Expiratory wheeze uncommon unless overt pulmonary oedema present	■ Crepitations ■ Peripheral oedema	■ Oedema rarely pitting unless cor pulmonale established ■ Normal JVP ■ Heart sounds soft, no murmurs ■ Crepitations are coarse and may vary with coughing ■ Expiratory wheeze common
Investigations	■ Spirometry normal ■ BNP significantly elevated in diuretic naive patients ■ ECG – often abnormal (left bundle branch block, evidence of anterior Q waves and poor R wave progression) ■ CXR – cardiomegaly and pulmonary congestion		■ Spirometry shows characteristic COPD pattern ■ BNP may be normal or mildly elevated ■ ECG – often normal, with large prominent p waves sometimes present if COPD is long standing ■ CXR – normal heart size, hyperinflated lungs, possible pneumonic change during exacerbations

Prescribing Points

1. **Effective use of long-acting nitrates**

   Long-acting nitrates lose their effectiveness if prescribed inappropriately. Most once-daily mononitrate preparations will last approximately 12 hours, but a nitrate-free period is needed to prevent tolerance developing, so twice-daily dosing should be avoided.

2. **Managing statin intolerance**

   Intolerance can be a major hurdle to prescribing, with muscle-related problems accounting for two-thirds of side effects. This can present early or late (sometimes years after initiation) and some agents – such as fibrates, macrolide antibiotics, calcium channel blockers and grapefruit juice – may exacerbate statin-related myopathy. A little statin is better than none, and very low-dose alternate days or even weekly regimes of rosuvastatin 5 mg can sometimes be tolerated and may bring about significant cholesterol reduction, particularly if combined with ezetimibe. There are now several alternative agents to statins including bempedoic acid, which can be used with ezetimibe in a fixed combination, as well as powerful injectable agents such as the PCSK9 inhibitors (alirocumab, evolocumab) and most recently inclisiran.

3. Using direct oral anticoagulants (DOACs) effectively

These have revolutionised anticoagulation therapy for stroke prevention in non-valvular atrial fibrillation (NVAF); however, there remains confusion over what constitutes NVAF. Valve-related atrial fibrillation, which precludes the use of DOACs, does not include all valvular pathology but is confined to mechanical prosthetic valves and patients with at least moderate mitral stenosis. DOACs have significant advantages over warfarin including a more consistent effect and a better safety profile, particularly in respect of intracranial haemorrhage.

4. Dual antiplatelet therapy – for whom and how long

The exponential growth of coronary stenting has been accompanied by evermore complex antiplatelet regimes. Implantation of a metal coronary stent requires early and effective antiplatelet therapy to prevent the devastating effects of stent thrombosis – so aspirin is combined with clopidogrel, ticagrelor or prasugrel. This combination is usually continued for up to 12 months, with discontinuation of the newer agent at that stage and lifelong aspirin as a monotherapy thereafter. All too often, patients are left on combination therapy indefinitely as a default, with an accompanying increased risk of haemorrhage with little further clinical benefit. Premature discontinuation to allow for surgery should be discussed with the cardiology team if possible.

5. Antiplatelets and anticoagulants

Around 10%–15% of patients undergoing coronary stenting will also have concurrent atrial fibrillation. Therapy to prevent stent thrombosis along with anticoagulants for stroke prevention creates a substantial bleeding risk in a population already at high baseline risk and therefore the need to restrict combination therapy to a minimum duration is paramount. The risk of stent thrombosis is highest in the first month and so most operators will anticipate combination therapy (two antiplatelet agents in addition to an anticoagulant) for the first 4 to 6 weeks, although depending on individual patient factors this may vary considerably and individual operators should provide instructions on discharge. Following this initial 'triple therapy period', one of the antiplatelet agents is dropped (usually aspirin) leaving of a single antiplatelet agent along with an anticoagulant for up to 12 months following the index procedure. Beyond this period, current guidelines support the use of an anticoagulant only without additional antiplatelet therapy. Outside of this indication, in an unstented coronary disease population, atrial fibrillation can be managed with an oral anticoagulant only without the need for an additional antiplatelet agent. It is imperative that combination therapy is under regular review, as all too often patients are left on potentially hazardous combinations beyond any clinical need. Clarification should always be sought on the duration of combination therapy where doubt exists.

CARE OF THE ELDERLY

James Woodard

Ten Pearls of Wisdom

1. **The absence of typical UTI symptoms in older patients means it probably isn't a UTI**
   … And isolated confusion is not a typical symptom, so it requires a full evaluation for other causes before a diagnosis of UTI can be made. Typical symptoms include new dysuria, frequency, urgency, suprapubic tenderness, polyuria or haematuria. Bear in mind, too, that the prevalence of asymptomatic bacteriuria – the presence of bacteria in the urinary tract of a patient without typical symptoms of a UTI – increases with age, institutionalisation and the presence of permanent catheters. This asymptomatic colonisation of the urinary tract means urine dips should be avoided as a diagnostic tool in older patients as the test is often positive even in the absence of an infection and their use leads to the overdiagnosis of UTIs.

2. **Delirium may well point to underlying dementia and so needs follow-up**
   Delirium is an acute state of confusion which fluctuates, results in an altered consciousness level and reduces levels of attention (see also the 'Easily confused' section). In up to 20% of patients, no cause is found, but it is not normal for older patients to become delirious. It should be considered a marker of lowered neurological reserve and is a good predictor of who will go on to develop dementia. One study has suggested that up to 60% of patients presenting to hospital with delirium but no known dementia diagnosis had dementia at a 3-month follow-up.

3. **The majority of older patients in the community are not frail – but know how to spot it**
   Frailty is a syndrome that is used to describe a group of mostly older patients who are vulnerable to a medical crisis as a result of minor illness, medication changes or other minimal stimuli.
   Individuals with frailty will often have a slower walking speed, decreased activity levels, muscle weakness, exhaustion and weight loss. Clinically, people

DOI: 10.1201/9781003304586-4

with frailty can be identified by electronic frailty screening tools or the Clinical Frailty Scale. The Clinical Frailty Scale defines frailty as a score from 1 to 9, 1 being fit and 9 being terminally ill. Day-to-day care should be determined by the clinical need of the patient, with the scores used to help plan services and distribute resources.

Patients with frailty will often be in care homes or need help with daily living activities, and many will have multiple comorbidities. Most older people in the community are not frail, however.

4. Recurrent falls are linked with dementia

Patients with dementia are twice as likely to fall when compared to cognitively intact individuals of the same age. They are also more likely to suffer recurrent falls, injure themselves or end up in care homes after the fall. The reasons for the increased risk of falls are numerous, but dementia likely affects both the balance centres of the brain and the patient's gait. If a patient is falling repeatedly or they have poor recall of the events, it is worth exploring their cognition alongside the appropriate referral to a multidisciplinary team falls clinic.

5. Life expectancy in care homes is lower than most people think

While some individuals live for many years in care homes, the average life expectancy of residents is much lower than you might imagine. People in residential care can expect to live on average for 2 years, while for those who need nursing care, survival drops to only 1 year. This has important implications, as current palliative care thinking is that we should be asking ourselves when considering advance care planning the following question: 'Is this patient at risk of dying within the next year?' Advanced care planning is time-consuming and challenging, but is vital in providing a comfortable and dignified end of life.

6. Beware of polypharmacy – ask yourself, 'Under these circumstances, would I take this medication?'

Problematic polypharmacy is the presence of multiple medications, some of which are inappropriate, potentially harmful or of no benefit.

Older patients are at greater risk of adverse drug reactions (ADRs), which make up a third of adverse events (AEs) relating to polypharmacy. These adverse events carry a significant morbidity and mortality risk. Evidence suggests 10%–30% of hospital admissions in the older population are associated with polypharmacy.

To complicate matters, these patients often benefit the most from careful prescribing. There are numerous checklists and guidelines available for medication reviews, but perhaps the best thing to do is ask yourself this question: Would I take that medication if I was in their situation? Your opinion and that of your patient are more important than non-individualised guidelines.

7. Ensure you clarify what patients mean when they complain of feeling dizzy

This is a problem seen in ENT clinics too (see the 'ENT' chapter). The clinician must identify exactly what the patient means. Broadly speaking, there are three categories.

a. *Vertigo*: A true sensation of spinning or significant movement. This is normally caused by problems in the vestibular system.

b. *Lightheadedness or syncope*: Feeling faint with the sensation they might black out. The cause is normally cardiovascular in origin.

c. *Unsteadiness*: A complex symptom of feeling of imbalance. Normally, this relates to a combination of problems of muscle strength, vestibular function, gait and posture.

8. Fracture risk should be assessed in all patients who fall

Bone mineral density decreases from the age of 35, with an associated increase in fractures in later life. Consequences of these potentially preventable fragility fractures range from chronic pain in vertebral fractures to 30% mortality within 1 year of a hip fracture. Anyone over the age of 65 years with a history of falls should have a fracture risk assessment done in primary care using either the FRAX score or QFracture calculator. However, both probably underestimate the fracture risk in older patients with recurrent falls. Treatment with bisphosphonates is very safe and effective, with side effects such as osteonecrosis of the jaw being extremely rare.

9. 24-hour tapes are rarely useful in falls assessments

Twenty-four-hour ECG recordings for falls are often inappropriately requested in primary and secondary care. In patients with a normal resting ECG, the pick-up rate for significant cardiac arrhythmias is only 1 or 2 per 100 24-hour tapes. In practice, unless there are red flag symptoms of syncope without warning, palpitations or chest pain, the cause is unlikely to be cardio-arrhythmic if the resting ECG is normal. A careful history, cardiac examination, and a proper lying and standing blood pressure are much more likely to reveal the cause of the fall.

10. Constipation in older people is common – but rectal examinations (PRs) are not

Constipation is extremely common in older people – relevant factors include fluid status, mobility, polypharmacy and changes in bowel motility. Constipation alone can cause delirium and agitation, so a PR examination is vital when assessing new confusion (see Pearl 1). Similarly, any patient found to be in painless, low-pressure urinary retention should have a PR and constipation treated before a catheter is inserted. Constipation also results in overflow diarrhoea, which is the most common cause of faecal incontinence. Again, a PR is needed to confirm this and then treatment with laxatives is required to stop this diarrhoea by removing the obstructive constipation.

Obscure or Overlooked Diagnoses

1. **Post-prandial hypotension (PPH)**

   This occurs in up to one-third of older patients. It is defined as a drop in systolic blood pressure greater than 20 mmHg when standing up following a meal. Lightheadedness, falls and syncope can occur up to 2 hours after eating. The reduction in blood pressure is a result of blood pooling in the abdomen to promote effective digestion of the meal. Certain conditions increase the risk of PPH in later life – including Parkinson's disease, diabetes and persistent hypertension. The risk is exacerbated by large, carbohydrate-heavy meals, warm temperatures and alcohol. Diagnosis is usually confirmed by a 24-hour blood pressure monitor and its correlation to symptoms.

   Treatment involves small regular meals and avoiding exacerbating factors. Advice about recognising the symptoms and sitting or lying down after meals should be given. Antihypertensives should be reviewed and, where possible, doses should be reduced, spread out or ideally stopped altogether.

2. **Carotid sinus syndrome (CSS)**

   This is a rare but significant cause of pre-syncope, syncope and falls in older people. It is very unusual in anyone under 50 years old. Patients complain of symptoms when the carotid baroreceptors are stimulated by movements such as turning the head, neck extension or wearing tight-fitting collars. CSS causes either a few seconds of asystole (requiring a pacemaker) or an episode of hypotension (treatment focusing on advice, hydration and reducing risk factors for low blood pressure). In patients with CSS who suffer falls, many will have no memory of episodes of loss of consciousness. This means they deny syncope, even though it was witnessed. It is often misdiagnosed as 'vertebrobasilar insufficiency', which is a clinical syndrome that doesn't exist.

3. **Normal pressure hydrocephalus (NPH)**

   This is caused by the abnormal build-up of cerebrospinal fluid within the cerebral ventricles. It results in a classic triad of symptoms of cognitive impairment, urinary incontinence and gait abnormalities. The disease is gradually progressive, with gait abnormalities and incontinence often presenting as early features. The gait is slow, broad-based and shuffling with the appearance of the feet sticking to the floor. Although it can progress more quickly than many dementia syndromes, it is potentially reversible with treatment. If the history is consistent with these symptoms, a CT head and neurology referral should be considered. The patient with NPH may benefit from a ventriculoperitoneal (VP) shunt.

Easily Confused

1. Parkinson's disease, depression and Alzheimer's dementia

	Parkinson's disease	Depression	Alzheimer's dementia
Cognitive decline	■ Late onset ■ Over 1 year after presence of motor symptoms	■ None in mild depression ■ Pseudo-dementia – presents as subacute decline that fluctuates with mood	■ Prominent feature ■ Progressive decline over years
Depressive symptoms	■ Common in later stages	■ Prominent feature in early stages	■ Common in later stages
Hallucinations	■ Not common ■ May be present in late disease	■ Not common ■ May be present in severe psychotic depression	■ Not common ■ May be present in late disease
Parkinsonism	■ Prominent feature ■ Normally unilateral at onset	■ Rarely found	■ Rarely found
Gait	■ Classic Parkinson's gait	■ Not affected unless depression very severe	■ Apraxic gait
Falls	■ Often not a feature at diagnosis but occur during disease progression	■ Not common	■ Occur later in the disease
Tremor	■ Common	■ Not present	■ Rare

2. Delirium and dementia

	Delirium	Dementia
Onset	■ Acute (days)	■ Slow (months)
Course	■ Fluctuating	■ Gradual deterioration
Awareness	■ Hyperactive = increased, agitated ■ Hypoactive = decreased, passive	■ Normal until later stages
Attention	■ Reduced	■ Normal until later stages
Memory	■ Poor working memory and recall	■ Poor short-term memory
Delusions	■ Short-lived and changeable	■ Fixed
Hallucinations	■ Transient visual hallucinations	■ Mixed hallucinations in later stages

3. Polymyalgia rheumatica (PMR) and osteoarthritis

	PMR	Osteoarthritis
Pain onset	■ Develops over days	■ Gradual onset over years
Pain characteristics	■ Ache and stiffness worse in the morning and often relieved by movement	■ Pain worse on movement with minimal morning pain or stiffness
Joint involvement	■ Generalised proximal muscles and joints (shoulder and thigh)	■ Normally affects a few large joints (knee, hip and spine)
Functional effects	■ Difficulty in washing and dressing in the morning	■ Restricted mobility due to lower limb joint pain
Inflammatory markers	■ CRP and ESR raised	■ Normal
Examination findings	■ Often normal examination	■ Joint deformity and pain common
Response to steroid therapy	■ Rapid improvement in days	■ No significant effect

Prescribing Points

1. **Antipsychotics in dementia**

   Antipsychotic medications have historically been overprescribed, despite their risks in older patients. Haloperidol or risperidone should only be prescribed for short courses in extreme cases and need to be regularly reviewed. This is because patients on antipsychotics have higher mortality than similar patients whose behaviour is managed non-pharmacologically. The higher death rates are secondary to an increased risk of stroke and transient ischaemic attacks (TIAs). Antipsychotics are also associated with an increased risk of falls, postural hypotension and temperature disturbances.

2. **Incontinence medications and dementia**

   Incontinence is common in patients with dementia. There are various reasons for this, including failure to recognise the need to void, failure to get to the toilet in time, communication problems and difficulty with undressing to use the toilet. Incontinence in patients with dementia is rarely solely secondary to detrusor instability, so the classic anticholinergic medications are unlikely to help. These treatments are associated with confusion and an increase in the rate of cognitive decline and therefore should be avoided in patients with dementia.

3. **ACE inhibitors and diuretics in acute illness – sick day rules**

   ACE inhibitors and diuretics are commonly prescribed in older patients. While there are many benefits to such therapies, both can exacerbate kidney injury and electrolyte imbalance in acute illness. Stopping such medications in patients with gastrointestinal symptoms similarly is vital; any condition that causes drowsiness and reduced oral intake should prompt cessation of these medications until 48 hours after the patient has recovered.

4. **Medication reviews for patients admitted to care homes**

    When patients are admitted to a care home they require a complete medication review. This is because they tend to be frail with multiple comorbidities and are therefore at high risk of polypharmacy, falls and adverse drug events. For example, it may be possible to stop antidepressant and antipsychotic medication. Also, many patients in care homes have a short life expectancy, so statins, ACE inhibitors, antihypertensives and other prognosis-improving medications may no longer be of benefit and should be reviewed on an individualised basis.

CHILDHOOD BEHAVIOURAL PROBLEMS

Wei Meng Chin

Ten Pearls of Wisdom

1. Include crucial information to avoid bounce-back when referring challenging behaviour

Challenging behaviour covers a range of behaviours including significantly frequent meltdowns or emotional dysregulation, aggression and violent behaviour. The high demand for services inevitably increases the threshold for acceptance of referrals. To reduce the risk of rejection and to help the receiving team direct the child and family to the correct service, try to include key information, such as:

- Details of physical aggression – such as punching, kicking and slapping people, or smashing furniture
- Information about verbal aggression – for example, calling names, swearing
- Frequency – sometimes, often or very often
- Duration – many services will only accept if problems have been present for 6 months or longer
- Triggers
- Impact – low, medium, high or at crisis point
- Strategies used so far
- Comorbidities – such as autism spectrum disorder (ASD), learning disability and global developmental delay

2. Consider autism in children presenting with anxiety

When a child presents with separation anxiety, social anxiety or school anxiety/refusal/phobia – or a combination of these – explore possible autism. Although these are not pathognomonic of ASD, they are quite common presentations or comorbidities in children with this problem. So try to identify any autistic features and refer for autism assessment as appropriate. If the severity of the anxiety is high, a referral to local mental health or psychology services is needed, sooner rather than later, for therapeutic input.

DOI: 10.1201/9781003304586-5

3. Autism is often associated with a delay in toileting skills

It is common for children with autism to experience a delay in the development of toileting skills. As a result, some may have to use nappies or pull-ups into adolescence or teenage years. The causes are multifactorial, including delay in understanding social contexts, impaired social self-care skills, sensory processing difficulties and ritualistic behaviour. This may result, for example, in a teenager who might only open her bowels in a pull-up in her bedroom, but not in the toilet. These situations can cause children and parents significant stress. While signposting to resources such as the ERIC website (https://eric.org.uk/) might be helpful, these skills tend to develop only when the child is ready – forcing the issue may simply add to the stress. The GP might consider referring to specialised behavioural services that support toileting in children with additional needs, if available, and when the child is older.

4. Developmental delay can be specific or global

Global developmental delay involves significant delay in at least two domains of developmental skills. Health visitors are the preferred referrers to developmental (community) paediatricians as their remit includes assessment, early intervention and monitoring. In the interim, a GP referral will be required if there is a need for a neurology or paediatric opinion over concerns of possible neurological or neuromuscular problems. Children with global developmental delay often have a risk of progressing to learning difficulties or disabilities later in life. Isolated delay in speech and language skills, without other neurological concerns, requires referral to a speech and language therapist and paediatric audiology (to rule out hearing impairment) but does not generally warrant a referral to paediatricians.

5. Do not refer children under 5 years of age for ADHD assessment

Boisterous (hyperactive), inattentive and impulsive behaviours are common (as normal variants) in children under 5, though these also may be early manifestations of ADHD. Only make a referral to specialist services if these symptoms persist beyond 5 years and include a report from the school and the parent. These children may present initially with restlessness, disruptiveness, anger issues or anxiety, but a referral should also detail key ADHD features such as the child having a short attention span, being easily distracted, disorganised and forgetful of daily routines, being fidgety and constantly on the go, and tending to interrupt others' conversations or activities. Simple helpful strategies that GPs can advise parents include simplifying instructions, breaking activities into chunks, using visual aids such as timetables, movement breaks (which allow the child to burn off energy and then refocus) and fidget toys.

6. Referrals to educational psychologists to assess possible learning disability should come from the school – though GP referral to paediatrics may be required, too

Learning disability, or intellectual disability, includes deficits in both cognitive ability and adaptive functioning. Cognitive or intellectual functioning is measured as IQ (intelligence quotient) and presents as difficulties in reasoning, judgement, problem-solving and learning from experience or teaching. Impairment in adaptive functioning includes difficulties in skills of daily life, social responsibility or independence, such as self-care skills (hygiene and preparing foods), managing money and social participation. When assessing possible learning disability, children should be referred to the appropriate service: educational psychologists. These referrals should be made directly by the relevant school, without involving the GP. The role of the GP is to refer to the paediatrician if a medical investigation for aetiology is needed, such as concerns regarding genetic conditions (such as Down's syndrome), hypothyroidism, neurometabolic conditions and so on.

7. Symmetrical clumsiness with no neuromuscular deficit may indicate developmental coordination disorder (DCD)

This was previously known as 'dyspraxia', and may present to the GP with:

- Clumsy hand–eye coordination
- Difficulty catching or throwing a ball
- Poor handwriting or cutting skills using scissors
- Difficulty in dressing, e.g. fastening zips or buttons
- Difficulty in maintaining hygiene, such as brushing teeth or wiping their bottom

Referral will result in a multidisciplinary assessment in which the paediatrician rules out neuromuscular causes such as Duchenne's neuromuscular disorder and the occupational therapist provides a detailed assessment of motor coordination and treatment.

8. Consider behavioural intervention and strategies in three tiers

Intervention for behaviour, emotional or mental health difficulties can usefully be considered in three tiers. Parents and schools can usually access Tier 1 and 2 services through self-referral or referral by teachers, respectively. The following illustrates this concept using autism as an example:

- Tier 1 often focuses on early intervention and prevention. Resources include charities (through workshops and parent support groups), online help, an individual educational plan at school and health visitors for those under 5 years old.
- Tier 2 includes targeted services such as educational psychologists, specialist advisory teachers, community counselling, mentoring at school and Tier 2 mental health services.

- GP may need to make referrals to Tier 3 mental health or psychology services specialising in autism support. The team and approach are usually multidisciplinary, including a psychologist, behaviour analyst, psychiatrist, social worker and family support worker. Management may require pharmacological treatment by psychiatrists.

9. ADHD medications do not treat autism or autism-related emotional dysregulation

Emotional dysregulation is difficulty in modifying or adapting emotions, resulting in a range of behaviours such as irritability, temper outbursts, meltdowns and aggression. Children with either ASD or ADHD are at risk of this. In children with ADHD, the cause is inattention to the emotional state and impulsivity, whereas children with ASD are at risk because of poor emotional awareness, difficulty in using emotional language, poor flexibility and high sensitivity to change. ADHD medication does not treat autistic features, or emotional dysregulation that is attributable to ASD. So for children with dual diagnoses of ASD and ADHD, while ADHD medications may ameliorate the challenges if ADHD predominates, there is no guarantee that this will be the case, especially if the emotions are more likely to be attributable to ASD (such as ritualistic behaviour, inflexibility with change and sensory differences). If ADHD specialists have optimised the child's medication, the GP could consider signposting or referring parents to Tier 3 services as described in Pearl 8.

10. Selective mutism is a form of speech anxiety or phobia

Selective mutism may present to the GP as an inability to speak consistently in certain social situations, such as school lessons or in public. It is not due to refusal to speak or speech and language difficulties. Affected children can, however, speak normally with a select few family members or familiar people in specific situations which they find comfortable. GPs should consider a referral to local paediatric mental health services if and when the issue leads to significant impairment of the child's functioning (such as education, family life and social communication). Treatment can include behavioural approaches (including individual play therapy, behavioural therapy and family therapy) and medication.

Obscure or Overlooked Diagnoses

1. Avoidant restricted food intake disorder (ARFID)

A limited diet is common in children with autism and some children with normal or typical development. Interventions include diversifying the child's diet, sensory strategies or a referral to a dietitian. When the symptoms become extreme or significant, avoidant restricted food intake disorder should be considered. This is a feeding disturbance characterised by a lack of interest in food or eating, avoidance associated with sensory features of the foods or concern about the consequences of aversive eating (such as choking or vomiting). To fulfil the diagnostic criteria, these features must be severe enough to cause one or more of the following:

- Significant weight loss
- Significant nutritional deficiency
- Dependence on enteral feeding or oral nutritional supplements
- Marked interference with psychosocial functioning

Children at increased risk of developing this disorder include those with autism spectrum disorder, anxiety disorder and a history of gastroesophageal reflux. Tertiary centres usually have strict criteria for referrals, ideally from developmental paediatricians or child and adolescent psychiatrists, so the GP suspecting this condition should refer using the local pathways as a first step.

2. Pathological (or extreme) demand avoidance (PDA)

This is not a diagnosis but a description of behaviour when children excessively avoid the demands of daily routines or tasks. It is often recognised as a 'PDA profile' in children with autism. Other additional characteristics may include obsession with other people (which may result in tricky relationships), excessive mood swings and impulsivity, and appearing excessively controlling and dominating, especially when feeling anxious. If it becomes extremely challenging and impairing at home and school, it requires referral to a highly specialised clinical psychology or mental health service. There is currently insufficient research data to indicate whether PDA could be present in the non-autism population.

3. Sensory processing difficulties

Sensory processing difficulties are not a diagnosis but a description of sensory-related behaviour that is excessively out of proportion for age. It could present as hyporeactivity (high pain threshold), hyperreactivity (such as clothing seams or labels making them feel itchy), sensory seeking (chewing objects) or sensory discrimination problems (difficulty interpreting specific sensory stimuli). Significant sensory differences (present in more than 90% of children with ASD) have been included in the diagnostic criteria of ASD. Studies in adults have highlighted that sensory differences are common in psychiatric disorders. The impact could range from mild to severe. The effectiveness of strategies differs from one child to another. Simple measures include ear defenders, a chewy necklace and so on. GPs can advise parents or carers to access strategies through official and reliable online resources. In severe cases, a referral or self-referral can be made to local sensory workshops or services, often run by occupational therapists.

Easily Confused

1. Motor tics and motor stereotypies

Motor tics	Motor stereotypies
■ Premonitory urge	■ No premonitory urge
■ Suppressible by the child, which can lead to feelings of dissatisfaction	■ Rarely voluntarily suppressed; may be suppressed by external distraction
■ Age of onset usually between 4 and 6 years	■ Age of onset usually before 3 years
■ Simple tics	■ Stereotypical movement or mannerisms
■ Eye blinking	■ Hand flapping or rotating
■ Shoulder shrugging	■ Flicking or twisting fingers
■ Nose or mouth twitching	■ Spinning oneself around
■ Tongue protrusion	■ Repeatedly bouncing up and down
■ Vocal tics	■ Head banging
■ Complex tics	■ Body rocking if combined with other complex movements
■ Copropraxia – a tic-like sexual or obscene gesture	■ Conditions
■ Echopraxia – a tic-like imitation of somebody else's movements	■ Primary motor stereotypies – in children with normal development
■ Conditions	■ Secondary stereotypies – in children with developmental or neurodevelopmental
■ Chronic motor tic disorder	problems. such as ASD, learning
■ Tourette's syndrome (chronic disorder of motor and vocal tic)	disabilities, sensory impairment, neurometabolic disorders

For all:
■ If mild to moderate, reassure, signpost to self-help courses, charities and online resources
■ Refer to specialised services for diagnosis and therapy, if they cause significant impairment or if GP is unsure and considers significant differential such as seizure

2. Truancy and school refusal

Truancy	School refusal
Unexcused, surreptitious, parents unaware	With parental knowledge
Non-anxiety based	Anxiety based (separation, generalised or social anxiety, or specific anxiety about aspect of schooling)
Linked to conduct disorder, academic problems, social issues and poverty	No such links
No real distress at prospect of going to school	Proposal of going to school causes severe distress
Uncommon in primary school children	Most common at starting school, changing classes or changing one school to another
No physical symptoms but may present with various mental health problems such as depression	May present to GP with physical symptoms

Prescribing Points

1. ADHD treatment

Children require six monthly measurements of weight (three monthly for those under 10), height, blood pressure and heart rate. This is to monitor potential side effects such as weight loss secondary to appetite suppression and altered blood pressure or heart rate.

Once the child has been stabilised on medication, paediatricians or child psychiatrists may use a clear monitoring plan to share care with the GP, who may then be able to help with monitoring and provide repeat prescriptions.

ADHD medications are contraindicated in those taking alcohol or recreational drugs.

2. Melatonin

There is a lack of evidence on the safety profile of melatonin use in sleep disorders in children, although experience suggests it can be used safely for children with problems such as ASD and ADHD. Theoretically, it should help with sleep onset difficulties. Modified release preparations can also help some children's maintenance of sleep. The aim is to reset the child's sleep rhythm. The standard advice is for a child to try it for 3 to 6 months followed by a washout period (trial without melatonin). Some children may no longer need the treatment, while others may need it longer term.

Shared care plans between GP and consultant may be used locally.

3. Medication for mental illness in children

GPs are well-versed in prescribing medication for common mental health problems in adults. However, children with mental health issues who may require medication need assessment by a child and adolescent psychiatrist. Responsibility for initiating medication and monitoring should also lie with the specialist.

CLINICAL BIOCHEMISTRY

Helen Ashby

Ten Pearls of Wisdom

1. **Make friends with your local laboratory – there is someone to help with clinical biochemistry conundrums**

   Clinical biochemistry covers a whole range of diseases from birth to death and everything in between. Some tests are done on site within your local lab and some will be sent away to central laboratories for specialised testing. Every lab has a duty biochemist (either a medic or a clinical scientist who is trained in biochemistry); they are experts in the way things are measured, problems with measuring and the method used, and interpretation of results. They are available to help you with patient care and can give advice on the next best investigation. So if in doubt about the way forward with abnormal biochemical blood tests, don't be afraid to seek help.

2. **Fit and healthy people can have 'abnormal' results**

   Reference ranges are worked out by laboratories testing a range of parameters in 'healthy' people, i.e. those who don't have any medical diagnosis or symptoms. The 95% confidence intervals are then taken as the 'normal' range (laboratory teams will always use reference range rather than normal range due to the implication of the word 'normal'). This means the lowest 2.5% and highest 2.5% of people who are not ill are classed as abnormal. Inevitably, then, when many parameters are checked in a patient, by default one may well be abnormal without the presence of disease. This highlights the importance of targeting testing according to the patient's disease/symptoms, otherwise, you may end up chasing results which are outside the reference range but of no clinical significance.

3. **Sample handling issues can lead to abnormal results**

   Pre-analytical factors (things that happen before the blood undergoes testing on the analyser) can have profound effects on results but are usually a diagnosis of hindsight. Blood tests in biochemistry can be contaminated by preservatives in other blood tubes, be affected by blood cells breaking up or have problems

DOI: 10.1201/9781003304586-6

because of the temperatures they are transported in. Laboratory scientists are usually good at looking out for and spotting these issues, but some are subtle and lead to the 'abnormal' results being reported to the GP. If the test is not in keeping with the patient's diagnosis, it is best to repeat it – treat the patient, not the result.

4. Know how to interpret hyponatraemia

Sodium is one of the most frequently requested tests from primary care, and abnormal results are common. Sodium is the major extracellular electrolyte and determines the water content of the body. Hyponatraemia is seen more commonly than hypernatraemia. Hyponatraemia can result from salt loss (genuinely low sodium level) or water excess (normal sodium level but watered down with too much fluid). So, to interpret low sodium, you need to know the patient's fluid status. If the patient has features of dehydration, the low sodium is usually caused by salt depletion – in which case there is usually too much fluid being lost from the body, such as through diarrhoea and vomiting, or from the kidneys (Addison's or diuretics). If, however, the patient is euvolaemic or oedematous, then it is likely to result from water overload. The latter is seen in oedematous states (heart failure, liver failure) or due to SIADH (see Pearl 5). Hyponatraemia is asymptomatic in many cases. Symptoms tend to occur when changes in the body's sodium levels are rapid, but these symptoms are non-specific (early symptoms include headache, nausea and weakness) and mimic other conditions.

5. Syndrome of inappropriate antidiuretic hormone (SIADH) is a common cause of hyponatraemia

SIADH is a diagnosis of exclusion and requires urine electrolytes and paired serum and urine osmolality to formally make the diagnosis. Also, all other causes of low sodium have to be excluded before the diagnosis can be made (renal failure, hypothyroidism, glucocorticoid deficiency and recent diuretic therapy). There are various medications which can cause SIADH, many of which are prescribed in primary care (see 'Prescribing points'). Other causes tend to be conditions which are located above the diaphragm (tumours, trauma and infection – the exception being pancreatic cancer, which tickles the bottom of the diaphragm). In SIADH, the body essentially 'holds on' to fluid and dilutes the body's sodium content; the low blood sodium causes the kidneys to stop excreting sodium. While urine is required for urinalysis, it can be difficult to get a paired osmolality sample; in a euvolaemic patient, low urea is suggestive of SIADH.

6. Hypercalcaemia may be spurious – repeat 'uncuffed' in mild to moderate cases

Hypercalcaemia is often discovered 'coincidentally' during 'routine' blood testing – this is certainly more common than finding a patient with symptoms of hypercalcaemia. If the hypercalcaemia is mild (2.6 mmol/L to 3.0 mmol/L), it may be the result of the tourniquet effect, and a repeat fasting uncuffed calcium may cause this to normalise. However, when repeating a check of calcium levels, vitamin D and PTH should also be requested, along with liver tests and renal profile. A detectable PTH in the presence of high calcium means likely hyperparathyroidism. This can occur with elevated calcium and a PTH in the reference range (as it should be suppressed by the high calcium). Phosphate is often low in hyperparathyroidism.

7. Timing can be everything

The timing of a biochemical test can have a significant effect on the result. For example, serum cortisol shows significant diurnal variation and so should be collected between 8 and 9 a.m. Similarly, testosterone peak levels occur in the early morning, with readings up to 50% lower in the evening – so testing should take place between 7 and 10 a.m. The menstrual cycle will affect hormone tests depending on when they are taken; progesterone should be assayed in the assessment of ovulation one week before the next anticipated period, which should correspond to the mid-luteal phase. Some timing effects can even be seasonal, with, for example, vitamin D levels being at their lowest towards the end of winter, and cholesterol being lowest in summer.

8. Know when an abnormal biochemical test is an emergency

Many of the more alarming biochemical tests may turn out to be spurious – but, of course, this is only something you can know in retrospect. As always, clinical decisions should be tempered by the presence (or not) of symptoms and how quickly the abnormality has developed (longer-standing and slowly developing abnormalities being less concerning). Severe hyperkalaemia (6.5 mmol/L or more) warrants immediate referral to secondary care; many GPs would feel most comfortable taking similar action with moderate levels (6.0–6.4 mmol/L), not least because the recommended urgent ECG might only be achievable via acute referral. In hyponatraemia, urgent secondary care advice should be sought if the level is below 125 mmol/L (or if below 130 mmol/L and symptomatic). Hypercalcaemia is probably the least common 'urgent' finding – a corrected level above 3.4 mmol/L warrants immediate referral.

9. Remember a biochemical work-up is needed in certain clinical situations

Keep biochemistry in mind in certain scenarios – it's easy to overlook. For example, sleep apnoea appears to have an association with type 2 diabetes, cardiovascular disease and non-alcoholic liver disease (NAFLD), so patients with this condition ought to have an assessment of cardiovascular risk parameters, liver function testing and HbA1c. Similarly, patients with polycystic ovary syndrome (PCOS) are at risk of metabolic disorders and so should have HbA1c and lipid profile measured – a pattern of the atherogenic lipoprotein phenotype is seen with low HDL cholesterol and high triglycerides. And gout is known to have an association with cardiovascular disease and so should have the appropriate biochemical work-up – plus an estimation of eGFR, as 25% of patients with gout also have CKD.

10. Don't stop thinking when HbA1c is normal in a patient with thirst – there could be another cause

In patients with thirst, diabetes mellitus is the first thing we – and patients – tend to think of. If the HbA1c/random blood sugar is normal, though, there's a temptation to assume the job is done. But there are other causes of thirst. Many are not 'biochemical', such as mouth breathing, anxiety, recent (especially spicy) food intake and medication side effects. But some are, including hypercalcaemia, CKD and diabetes insipidus. So in the genuinely and persistently thirsty patient in whom diabetes mellitus has been excluded, check plasma calcium, eGFR and serum/urine osmolality (plasma osmolality is high and urine osmolality low in diabetes insipidus; in another differential, compulsive water drinking, the plasma osmolality is usually low).

Obscure or Overlooked Diagnoses

1. Hypopituitarism

Hypopituitarism is often insidious in onset and diagnosis in primary care requires a high degree of suspicion for it to be recognised. The symptoms differ from patient to patient depending on which hormone is affected the most and how quickly the disease develops. Tiredness, weight gain, muscle weakness, change in body hair, dry skin and constipation are all symptoms, which can fit with many other conditions. Screening tests within laboratories for thyroid disease are usually with a thyroid-stimulating hormone (TSH), which may miss a pituitary condition, and therefore if this is suspected in a patient, then a specific request for pituitary thyroid hormones needs to be made to ensure appropriate testing.

2. Secondary causes of hypertension

Usual laboratory testing for hypertension involves checking for some common causes and consequences, such as assessing the end organs to ensure there is no damage and to ensure there are no complications from treatment. However, in some cases, screening for secondary hypertension is required (5%–10% of patients are thought to have an underlying cause). In young adults (usually those under 45 years of age) it is important to consider structural and endocrine causes of hypertension such as Cushing's syndrome (easy bruising may be the first sign), primary aldosteronism and phaeochromocytoma. First-line investigations would include renal function and urinalysis, the aldosterone–renin ratio, a renal ultrasound to assess kidney size, and, if there is clinical suspicion, 24-hour urine testing for catecholamines or metanephrines. However, plasma metanephrines are becoming more widely used due to the difficulties in the accurate collection of 24-hour urines, so it is best to contact the local laboratory to see which service is offered. Some laboratories use a two-stage testing strategy, with urine as an initial screen and then, if there are any doubts, moving onto blood taking as a second line.

3. **Addison's disease**

Addison's is known as a 'master of disguise', as it can mimic so many other pathologies. It is rare, affecting about 1:10,000, and many of its symptoms are very non-specific, hence diagnosis often being delayed. Features include tiredness, muscle weakness and pain, gastrointestinal disturbance, hyperpigmentation and dizziness via hypotension. One clue is the presence of other autoimmune problems such as coeliac disease or vitiligo. Biochemical analysis may reveal hyponatraemia and hyperkalaemia (though both can be normal) and a low early morning cortisol, though this lacks sensitivity, so specialist testing (such as a synacthen test) is required if the level of suspicion is high.

Easily Confused

1. True hyperkalaemia and pseudohyperkalaemia

Parameter	Hyperkalaemia	Pseudohyperkalaemia
Renal function	Often abnormal but not exclusively so	Likely normal or no change from previous
White cell count	Likely normal	May be raised (intracellular potassium released in vitro)
Platelet count	Likely normal	May be raised (intracellular potassium released in vitro)
Other biochemical tests	Other tests fit with possible disease state	If cause is contamination, then low alkaline phosphatase, low calcium levels (due to EDTA contamination from the full blood count tube)
Transport conditions	Satisfactory	More likely if sample has been exposed to extremes of heat, especially cold temperatures (or stored in fridge overnight)
Delay in separation	Satisfactory	Time of collection to time of receipt in lab >6 hours
Repeat test	Same result	Different (normal) result

2. Cushing's syndrome and simple obesity

Parameter	Cushing's syndrome	Simple obesity
Exogenous corticosteroids	Likely	Unlikely
Distribution of fat	Buffalo hump, moon face, thin legs	Uniform distribution
Other features	Proximal myopathy, marked striae, thin skin, facial plethora, easy bruising	Absent, although striae can be seen in simple obesity
Onset and progression	May be recent onset; progressive	Long term; may be progressive
Biochemical evidence of elevated cortisol	Present	Absent

Prescribing Points

1. Corticosteroid use

Short courses of corticosteroids (less than 3 weeks) can be stopped abruptly unless taken in high doses (more than 40 mg/day of prednisolone for more than a week). To avoid an 'Addisonian crisis', patients on long-term steroids should be warned never to stop them abruptly, given a steroid card and advised about 'sick day rules' – steroids may need to be increased in dose in acute illness to prevent an acute crisis. Mild illness without fever usually does not require a change in dose, but illness with fever in patients who are on prednisolone doses of less than 15 mg per day may require additional steroid medication. The same goes for a patient with vomiting and diarrhoea. In severe illness, patients should seek medical advice and an increased dose of steroids (e.g. prednisolone 20 mg) should be advised.

2. Sick day rules for patients at risk of acute kidney injury (AKI)

In patients at risk of AKI, sick day rules should be given for illnesses such as vomiting and diarrhoea, and fever with sweating and shaking. In these patients, non-steroidal anti-inflammatory medications, drugs that lower blood pressure and drugs which accumulate in patients with reduced kidney function should be avoided. These include diuretics and ACE inhibitors, metformin (which can lead to lactic acidosis) and those which may cause hypoglycaemia (such as sulfonylureas). Care should be exercised with trimethoprim, which can increase potassium and also interferes with creatinine secretion, giving a 'false positive' AKI.

3. Thyroxine dose changes

If making a change in a dose of thyroxine, the minimum time interval, assuming good compliance, is 4 weeks before there will be a change in the steady state of TSH (thyroxine treatment aims to maintain the TSH within the reference range unless a patient is pregnant, when it needs to be in the lower half of the reference range).

4. **Drug-induced biochemical abnormalities**

Always keep medications in mind when dealing with some of the commoner biochemical abnormalities. For example, hyperkalaemia may be caused by ACE inhibitors, A2RAs and potassium-sparing diuretics, and hypokalaemia by thiazide and loop diuretics. The possible list of medications that can be implicated in SIADH is very long and includes thiazides, SSRIs, PPIs, carbamazepine, tricyclics and phenothiazines. Thiazide diuretics can lead to hypercalcaemia, and fibrates can cause a reduction in eGFR, although this is not a true reduction – it is thought to be related to how the renal tubule handles creatinine when a fibrate is taken.

DERMATOLOGY

David Rutkowski, Zak Shakanti,
Minal Singh and Matthew Harries

Ten Pearls of Wisdom

1. Always perform a complete skin examination on dermatology patients

Approximately 20% of melanomas and 15% of cutaneous squamous cell carcinomas are missed due to incomplete skin examination by the first-contact practitioner in the UK. This usually occurs when the examination focus is solely on the presenting lesion, a tempting proposition when time is short. In fact, a recent World Health Organization report on diagnostic error in primary care highlighted the second commonest error rate among all cancer subtypes was in skin. Skin examinations also afford a crucial opportunity to promote skin health through skin cancer risk assessment and safe sun exposure advice. For example, counting moles on one arm can be used as a proxy for the total number of moles. Those with more than 11 moles on one arm are likely to have more than 100 moles on their entire skin, which is a known risk factor for melanoma. Those with very fair skin that easily burns are at a higher risk of actinic damage and non-melanoma skin cancer. Numerous leaflets are now available to support these health promotion activities (e.g. available from Cancer Research UK).

2. Use dermoscopy to recognise common benign lesions

Dermoscopy uses skin surface microscopy to eliminate surface reflection for a clearer view of a lesion. It is particularly useful in identifying benign lesions that do not require further investigation or referral. We would advise focusing on the identification of three frequently referred lesions as a good starting point. These are seborrheic keratoses, haemangiomas and subungual haematomas. Seborrheic keratoses show cribriform surface changes, milia-like cysts and comedo-like openings; haemangiomas display typical (red) lacunae; and subungual haematomas display the red-purple colour of the haemorrhage under the nail plate with small blood spots seen at the periphery of the discolouration. DermNet provides useful dermoscopic photos for comparison (see 'skin lesions, tumours and cancers' at dermnetnz.org). Identifying these common benign lesions will prevent patients from going through unnecessary worry in skin lesion clinics and

DOI: 10.1201/9781003304586-7

reduce referrals by at least 20%, offering improved capacity for those who most require specialist input.

3. A clear history, examination findings and good-quality photos are the key to effective remote consultations in dermatology

Remote consultations, teledermatology, and advice and guidance services are being used to streamline referrals and provide dermatology advice in a timely manner. Remote consultations are most beneficial when the diagnosis is already confirmed. A major pitfall in dermatological remote consultation is the inability to examine the skin. This confers considerable disadvantage to the clinician, as important pathophysiological changes that improve diagnostic accuracy are not accessible. Problems include the inability to palpate the skin (to determine which layer of skin is involved), poor appraisal of a lesion in the context of lesions elsewhere on the skin (e.g. the 'ugly duckling' sign describes a lesion that looks different to the rest, potentially representing a cancerous change) and inability to examine other areas that would help to support or refute the diagnosis. Success in teledermatology and advice and guidance services is dependent on two major factors.

- A thorough and detailed patient assessment. This should include, when appropriate, a complete skin cancer risk factor assessment and any examination findings that cannot be assessed via the accompanying 2-D imaging.
- Provision of good quality photographic images. These images need to be in focus and taken in good lighting, with the area of concern in the centre of the photograph. Both close-up and wider views help understand the location (for lesions) and pattern of presentation (for rashes), and inclusion of a size comparator (e.g. ruler) can also be helpful. Additional images may be required.

4. Control itch in eczema by treating the underlying inflammation, checking compliance and considering short-term sedating antihistamines

Pruritus in eczema can be difficult to manage. Ultimately, control of chronic pruritus is achieved by treating the underlying inflammation. Therefore, this is an opportune time to review the topical treatment regimen and address patient compliance with topical steroids, emollients and soap substitutes. The conventional use of non-sedating antihistamines is rarely effective, although sedating antihistamines may help (mainly due to their sedative effects), particularly during acute exacerbations where a short course may break the nocturnal 'itch–scratch' cycle. Daytime use is rarely needed.

5. Remember infection as a factor in skin conditions

Skin infections are common and may cause skin disease or complicate pre-existing disorders. For example, staphylococcal nasal carriage can predispose to recurrent exacerbations of eczema or folliculitis. When there is a sudden deterioration in eczema associated with localised pain and systemic upset, consider eczema herpeticum (i.e. superadded herpes virus infection) characterised by multiple vesicles that quickly burst leaving monomorphic crateriform lesions on the skin. Fungal skin infection inappropriately treated with topical steroids will show initial improvement then subsequent deterioration, with treatment changing the appearance (hence the term 'tinea incognito'); send skin scrapings to microbiology in packaging shielded from sunlight (fungal organisms are destroyed by UVB, increasing the likelihood of false negative results) in presumed 'dermatitis' unresponsive to steroid creams.

6. Most skin itch without a rash is benign

An itch without skin rash is very common and often transient; however, it can cause significant distress to the patient and result in poor sleep. Most cases are due to skin dryness, which becomes more common with increasing age and the use of harsh skin cleansers. Initial management is with avoidance of irritants (soaps, shower gels, bubble baths), the use of a soap substitute and regular applications of emollients. In those who do not settle, further investigation may be required to exclude an underlying cause (e.g. iron deficiency, thyroid dysfunction, liver disease, renal failure or underlying malignancy).

7. Do not underestimate the psychological impact of skin disease

Many skin disorders cause a reduction in quality of life, generate psychological distress and have a negative impact on relationships. Underlying reasons include the visual appearance of the condition, the reaction of the public to the patient's appearance (e.g. fears of contagion), functional effects (e.g. inability to work with chronic hand eczema) and the symptoms caused. Chronic skin conditions can have a profound effect on life choices and employment opportunities. Even when the condition is localised, it can still have a marked impact on an individual, particularly if there is involvement of the face, hands or genital skin. Recognition and acknowledgement are the first steps, with many potentially benefiting from professional psychological support.

8. IgE blood testing is rarely useful in paediatric eczema

Many parents ask whether their child's eczema is 'allergic' and may demand testing to various foods. Performing untargeted IgE tests to multiple foods is rarely helpful and should only be performed by those who are able to interpret the results. Positive results are commonly seen (70%–80%) and correlate poorly with how much the potential allergen contributes to the child's dermatitis. In general, if there is significant suspicion that certain foods exacerbate their eczema or the child has other symptoms to suggest a food allergy, a food diary is probably the most useful initial investigation. Caution is required when restricting a child's diet – seek input from a paediatric dietician. Patch testing for allergic contact dermatitis can sometimes be more helpful (see Pearl 9).

9. Don't forget contact allergy, especially in treatment-resistant patients

Allergic contact dermatitis is common. Most patients recognise their allergy (e.g. reactions to cheap jewellery indicating nickel allergy); however, unrecognised contact allergy may worsen known dermatoses and should be considered in treatment-resistant patients. They can be identified using patch testing. Certain areas of the skin are more prone to contact allergy. For example, any persistent predominantly facial or hand eczema warrants patch testing. Also, lower legs (e.g. treatment for leg ulcers) and peri-anal skin are prone to developing reactions.

10. If patients don't improve, consider an alternative diagnosis or inadequate treatment

If your patient does not improve after initial treatment, reassess and consider if the original diagnosis was correct. Skin disease commonly evolves over time, so diagnostic features might become apparent which were not present originally. Consider, too, whether the treatment offered was adequate. Common examples include courses of oral antibiotics for acne that are too short (assessing effectiveness usually requires 3 to 4 months of continuous use) or topical steroids that are insufficiently potent (e.g. a mild topical corticosteroid for chronic hand eczema in an adult, where a potent or super-potent corticosteroid is usually required).

Obscure or Overlooked Diagnoses

1. Stevens–Johnson syndrome/toxic epidermal necrolysis

These are rare, life-threatening mucocutaneous drug reactions occurring 2 to 4 weeks after drug exposure. Patients present with prodromal symptoms and skin pain followed by the development of dusky confluent erythema, target lesions, and widespread epidermal blistering and skin detachment. Common culprits include allopurinol, carbamazepine, lamotrigine, phenytoin, sulphur antibiotics and NSAIDs. These patients require emergency admission.

2. Cutaneous vasculitis

This is a group of conditions resulting from inflammation of blood vessels within the skin. The most common type seen in dermatology is cutaneous small vessel vasculitis presenting with palpable, non-blanching purpura predominantly affecting the lower limbs, which may ulcerate. Most are idiopathic, but infections, (autoimmune) inflammatory diseases, medication or underlying malignancy are other causes. Note that cutaneous vasculitis may be the initial presentation of a systemic vasculitis, so assess blood pressure, renal function and urine dipstick in all patients. An urgent dermatology review is recommended.

3. Scabies

Scabies usually presents with significant skin itch, particularly at night or after a bath or shower. Always enquire about itchy close ('touching') contacts, as others may also be infected. The skin may show various types of rashes, usually non-specific excoriations or eczema changes, and scabies burrows may be visible on the finger webs, wrists, ankles, nipples and genitals. Inflammatory papules on the penis of an itchy male should be regarded as scabies until proven otherwise. Despite successful treatment, patients may still complain of pruritus for up to 4 weeks afterwards. This does not necessarily represent treatment failure, just a settling allergic response to the infestation; a mild/moderate topical steroid may help here.

4. Erythroderma

Erythroderma is defined as confluent erythema of the skin covering over 90% of the body surface area. The main causes of erythroderma are eczema, psoriasis, pityriasis rubra pilaris, drug reactions, idiopathic erythroderma and lymphoma. Consequences of erythroderma include poor temperature and fluid regulation, loss of skin barrier function, dehydration, hypotension and high-output cardiac failure. Erythroderma is often well tolerated in younger patients but can be life-threatening in the elderly or those with significant comorbidities. Supportive treatment with bed rest, greasy emollients and fluid support is usually the initial approach to management. Hospital admission may be required.

5. Angioedema without wheals

Angioedema is commonly associated with cutaneous urticaria; however, when patients present with angioedema without skin wheals, it is important to consider drug causes (especially NSAIDs and ACE inhibitors) and C1 esterase deficiency. Initial investigation should include complement levels – low C4 is seen in C1 esterase deficiency and should prompt confirmatory tests (i.e. C1 esterase levels).

Easily Confused

1. Fungal nail disease/onychomycosis and psoriatic nail disease

Fungal nail disease/onychomycosis	Psoriatic nail disease
■ Nails are thickened, discoloured and brittle	■ Nails usually not friable
■ Mostly affects single/small number of toenails, usually asymmetrical	■ Mostly affects multiple fingernails in a symmetrical pattern; nail pitting, onycholysis and subungual hyperkeratosis
■ No features of psoriasis elsewhere on the skin; look for associated tinea pedis/other fungal infections	■ Psoriasis elsewhere on the skin; family history of psoriasis

2. Vitiligo and pityriasis alba

Vitiligo	Pityriasis alba
■ Any age ■ Completely depigmented patches with distinct borders with no inflammation or scale ■ Symmetrical distribution ■ May be poliosis (white hairs) ■ Has associations with other autoimmune conditions ■ No seasonal variation ■ Exhibits Koebner phenomenon	■ Seen in children between 3 and 16 years of age ■ Usually facial but can affect the neck, arms, and shoulders; can be mildly pruritic; generally, starts as an erythematous patch which develops a fine scale and then progresses to a smooth hypopigmented patch, which can become confluent ■ Seen in darker skin types or following sun exposure ■ Exact cause unknown but probably a form of atopic dermatitis ■ Generally, affects patients more in the summer months ■ No Koebner phenomenon

3. Alopecia areata and trichotillomania

Alopecia areata	Trichotillomania
■ Non-scarring ■ Sudden onset of hair loss and increased hair fall; any hair-bearing area can be affected; well-demarcated oval patches of hair loss with no visible inflammation; exclamation mark hairs may be seen ■ Positive pull test along the edge of the patches ■ Autoimmune associations	■ Self-inflicted damage to the hair (the patient may not acknowledge this as the cause) ■ Irregular 'bizarre looking' patches of alopecia ■ Variable length stubble in affected areas ■ Dermoscopy shows fractured hair shafts ■ Negative pull test ■ May reflect a significant underlying psychiatric pathology

4. Chondrodermatitis nodularis helicis and non-melanoma skin cancer

Chondrodermatitis nodularis helicis	Non-melanoma skin cancer
■ Inflammation of the ear cartilage (skin not involved) ■ Very tender nodule with central crust (crust = dried serous fluid) on the most prominent part of the ear – 'pointing outwards' ■ In men = helix; in women = antihelix more common ■ Patients prevented from sleeping on that side ■ Treatment: Pressure reduction and topical corticosteroids; surgical excision may be required	■ Neoplasm of the epidermal layer of the skin ■ Nodule with variable degrees of scale (scale = keratinocytes) ■ Usually on the top of the ear ■ May be tender ■ Treatment: surgical excision

Prescribing Points

1. **Topical corticosteroids**
   a. Children generally require less potent steroids than adults.
   b. In adults, treatment of the face and skin creases is usually limited to mild/moderate steroids; the trunk and limbs may require moderate-potency steroids; and the scalp, hands and feet often require more potent steroids.
   c. Certain conditions require more potent steroids (e.g. discoid lupus, lichen simplex).
   d. To gain patient confidence, consider applying a more potent steroid initially to attain control and then step down to a weaker agent.
   e. Prescribe adequate volumes. For example, an adult man will require 20 g each application to cover their entire skin surface.
   f. Consider using fingertip units (FTUs) to guide how much topical steroid to apply. An FTU is the amount of steroid cream that stretches from the tip to the distal finger crease of an adult index finger. One FTU is approximately 0.5 g and will cover the equivalent of two 'flat hands' (where the fingers are extended).
   g. Always apply topical treatments in the direction of hair growth to reduce the risk of folliculitis.

2. **Good emollient care is vital**
   Unfortunately, patients generally underutilise their moisturisers. Many patients will refuse repeated application of thick greasy emollients, so creams or lotions in the morning and a greasy emollient in the evening may be a reasonable compromise. The key is regular application, so the patient needs to like the product to use it. In general:
   a. Ointments are better than creams for very dry skin.
   b. Creams are better for weepy skin as it 'sticks' better.
   c. Avoid aqueous cream as a leave-on emollient (although it can be used as a soap substitute); it has been shown to reduce skin barrier function.
   d. Prescribe sufficient volumes. An adult will generally require more than 600 g per week.
   e. If someone is unsure how much to apply, advise them to apply enough to make the skin look shiny.

3. **Treatments for actinic keratosis**
   Actinic keratoses lesions are graded: 1 = slight erythema with the texture of fine sandpaper on palpation; 2 = palpable with scale; 3 = hyperkeratotic lesion or nodule. Evidence suggests that grade 3 lesions, and more than ten grade 1, 2 or 3 lesions in one area (field change) increase the risk of progression to cutaneous squamous cell carcinoma. Single grade 1 or grade 2 lesions do not carry this risk and can spontaneously regress, so conservative treatment with emollients alone

may be sufficient. Treatment for actinic keratoses aims to reduce progression to squamous cell carcinoma. Only Efudix® (5-fluorouracil) cream and Aldara® (5% imiquimod) cream achieve this. Solaraze® (diclofenac) gel does not and therefore is not cost-effective. The side effects of Efudix® (5-fluorouracil) cream and Aldara® (5% imiquimod) cream can cause moderate to severe inflammation, so patients need to be counselled about this reaction at treatment outset. Consider co-prescribing a mild-to-moderate topical corticosteroid for severe reactions.

4. **Hand care advice**

   Management of hand dermatitis includes avoidance of irritants, hand protection for manual work (cotton gloves for dry work/cotton-lined rubber gloves for wet work), soap substitutes for cleansing and regular applications of emollients. Consider prescribing smaller emollient sizes to enable the patient to carry the product at work or out and about.

5. **Never use trimethoprim in patients on methotrexate**

   Trimethoprim and methotrexate should never be prescribed concomitantly owing to the risk of life-threatening organ toxicity, particularly in patients with renal or hepatic impairment. Caution is required, as most dermatology patients have their methotrexate prescribed via the hospital, so it may not appear on the repeat prescription list.

DIABETES

Tahseen A. Chowdhury

Ten Pearls of Wisdom

1. **Try to distinguish between type 1 (T1D) and type 2 diabetes (T2D)**

   Distinguishing between T1D and T2D can be difficult. T1D may not conform to the usual stereotype, and T2D is now common in younger adults and children, particularly in high-risk ethnic populations. The following may help in distinguishing between T1D and T2D:

   a. Acute onset in a young, slim White European is most likely to be T1D. Conversely, non-White ethnicity, abdominal obesity or acanthosis nigricans suggests T2D.

   b. Significant ketonaemia or ketonuria is likely to indicate insulin deficiency associated with T1D.

   c. About 90% of people with T1D will have positive glutamic acid decarboxylase (GAD), zinc transporter-8 (ZnT8) or islet antigen-2 (IA-2) antibodies.

   d. Low levels of C-peptide (ideally checked post-prandially along with plasma glucose) in the presence of hyperglycaemia are more suggestive of T1D.

2. **People with T2D may develop diabetic ketoacidosis**

   Conventional teaching suggests that a person who develops diabetic ketoacidosis (DKA) must have T1D. There is, however, a subset of patients who develop DKA who have T2D. This condition is known as 'ketosis-prone T2D' and appears to be more common among African Caribbeans. The patient presents with typical DKA, but subsequently, insulin requirements drop and many patients are able to cease insulin. This condition should be considered in all patients presenting with DKA, in whom insulin requirements diminish rapidly (although this may be seen in T1D in the 'honeymoon period'). Negative diabetes antibodies should be confirmed, and the presence of elevated C-peptide also suggests some beta cell functional capacity. Insulin should be weaned very slowly, and then replaced with oral hypoglycaemics, typically starting with metformin.

DOI: 10.1201/9781003304586-8

Also, remember that the use of sodium-glucose transporter-2 inhibitors can sometimes cause euglycaemic DKA (see 'Prescribing points').

3. Know when you can't rely on glycated haemoglobin (HbA1c)

HbA1c is a useful test, with a level of 48 mmol/mol (6.5%) or above being diagnostic of diabetes (two tests in asymptomatic patients). But there are important caveats. Recent onset (<4 weeks) of acute symptoms necessitates the use of glucose tests in the diagnosis of diabetes, as the HbA1c may not have had sufficient time to rise. Conditions affecting red cell turnover, such as haemoglobinopathies, may affect the interpretation of HbA1c. More acute blood loss is likely to lower HbA1c owing to increased red cell turnover, while chronic iron deficiency may falsely elevate HbA1c due to reduced red cell turnover. In circumstances where HbA1c may not be suitable for monitoring diabetes, self-monitoring of blood glucose may have to be undertaken or the use of serum fructosamine (a glycated protein giving an estimate of glucose control over about 2 weeks) may be considered.

4. Think about pancreatic cancer in an older person presenting acutely with weight loss and hyperglycaemia

Diabetes is a risk factor for breast, liver, pancreatic and colon cancers. Cancer screening guidelines suggest that in a person presenting with diabetes and weight loss over the age of 60, pancreatic cancer should be considered.

5. Intervention in someone with pre-diabetes might dramatically reduce their risk of developing diabetes in the future

Individual interventions to reduce the risk of progression to diabetes in people at high risk are proven to be effective. In people with impaired glucose tolerance or pre-diabetes (HbA1c 42–47 mmol/mol), intervention to achieve a 5%–10% weight loss can reduce the risk of progression to diabetes by around 58%. The use of metformin is also proven to reduce the risk of progression to diabetes.

6. Avoid causing treatment-induced hypoglycaemia in older people

Hypoglycaemia is an important cause of morbidity in older people with T2D, being associated with falls, cardiovascular events, impaired cognition and poor quality of life. Tight glycaemic control in older people with T2D may not reduce the risk of complications, especially in patients with multiple comorbidities, so avoid overtreatment. This is reflected in various diabetes guidelines, which suggest individualisation of glycaemic targets – an HbA1c target of 75 mmol/mol may be perfectly suitable for an older person. Patients at risk of hypoglycaemia include those with chronic kidney disease stage 3 and below, those treated with insulin or sulfonylurea, and those with HbA1c <53 mmol/mol. In such patients, consider reducing hypoglycaemic agents.

7. Discuss and document car driving and diabetes

All drivers with diabetes treated with tablets or insulin should inform their insurance company and the DVLA. In patients on insulin or sulfonylureas, drivers should be advised to test blood glucose before driving and every 2 hours while driving. They should be aware of the symptoms of hypoglycaemia and how to treat them and should carry fast-acting glucose at all times when driving. Patients should report any instances of hypoglycaemia requiring third-party assistance. Two such episodes in 1 year will necessitate cessation of driving for 1 year. People who drive for a living will need to keep glucose records in a meter that is able to store at least 3 months of tests.

8. Be aware of the effects of travel on diabetes

Overseas travel poses problems for people with diabetes, particularly those on insulin. Confusion over the timing of insulin or drug therapy and meals can lead to problems with hyper- or hypoglycaemia. General advice should include advising their airline they have diabetes, carrying a letter confirming their need for insulin and sharps, and storing insulin in hand luggage. Patients should be advised about the possibility of more rapid insulin absorption due to greater physical activity or hot weather, which may increase the risk of hypoglycaemia. While travelling, blood glucose testing is needed every 4 to 6 hours. Eastward travel shortens the day and may require a reduction in insulin dose, while for westward travel the opposite applies.

9. Prioritise blood pressure and cholesterol when faced with multiple issues to manage

While glucose control is important to reduce the risk of diabetes microvascular complications, vascular complications are the main causes of mortality and morbidity in patients with diabetes. NICE guidelines suggest aiming for a blood pressure less than 140/90 mmHg in all people with diabetes, and 130/80 mmHg with cardiovascular disease or renal disease. Statin therapy should be offered to all people with T2D with a calculated 10-year cardiovascular risk of greater than 10%. In patients with T1D, statin therapy should be 'considered' in all and 'offered' in the presence of additional cardiovascular risk factors, nephropathy, for those over 40 years old or for those diagnosed with diabetes more than 10 years ago.

10. Depression is common among people with diabetes

Depression is an often overlooked diagnosis in people with diabetes. It is well recognised that depression can exacerbate diabetes, making it more difficult to control. Recognition and treatment of depression in people with diabetes may improve glucose control and quality of life.

Obscure or Overlooked Diagnoses

1. **Charcot neuroarthropathy**
   This is a diagnosis not to be missed. Patients frequently have long-standing peripheral neuropathy and present with a unilateral painless, swollen, warm foot. The condition often follows minimal trauma and may be mistaken for cellulitis or deep vein thrombosis. Pulses are usually easily felt and there are clinical signs of peripheral neuropathy. There is progressive instability and loss of joint function, ultimately leading to major deformity. Early recognition and referral are vital, as stabilisation of the joint is mandatory and can lead to significantly reduced morbidity.

2. **Autoimmune polyendocrine syndromes**
   T1D may be associated with a number of autoimmune endocrine conditions. In a person with T1D and a new onset of hypoglycaemia, hypoadrenalism (Addison's disease) or adult coeliac disease should be considered.

3. **Small intestinal bacterial overgrowth (SIBO)**
   Patients with diabetes are more prone to developing SIBO if they have diabetic gastroparesis, leading to nausea, vomiting and early satiety. Disordered peristalsis can lead to stasis of material within the small intestine, causing SIBO. Typical symptoms include nausea, bloating, vomiting, diarrhoea and weight loss. Gastroenterological expertise should be sought; treatment with rotating antibiotics and probiotics may help.

4. **Exocrine pancreatic insufficiency**
   While chronic pancreatitis is a well-recognised cause of diabetes, there appears to be an important association between diabetes and exocrine pancreatic insufficiency, with some studies suggesting it is surprisingly common (reported to be in about 25% of patients with diabetes). The resulting malabsorption may lead to weight loss, vitamin deficiencies, diarrhoea and bloating. Faecal elastase is a reasonable screening test.

5. **Monogenic diabetes**
   About 1% of diabetes diagnoses may be 'monogenic diabetes', such as 'maturity-onset diabetes in the young' (MODY). MODY is an important condition to consider, as treatment will vary according to its genetic subtype. MODY should be considered in patients with a strong family history of diabetes, typically diagnosed at under the age of 25. GADA and ICA are negative, and patients often have a reasonable production of C-peptide. The patient should be referred to a hospital diabetes clinic for consideration for genetic testing.

6. **Mitochondrial diabetes**
   Maternally inherited diabetes and deafness (MIDD), or mitochondrial diabetes, occurs due to a genetic defect in mitochondrial DNA, which is only inherited from maternal DNA. Most patients present with acute hyperglycaemia due to

insulin deficiency and hence are often labelled T1D. Lifelong insulin therapy is the norm owing to insulin deficiency. Sensorineural deafness occurs in about 75% of patients and pigmentary retinal changes may be seen. In a person with T1D and deafness, mitochondrial diabetes should be considered, as it may have implications for offspring.

7. **Lipohypertrophy of injection sites**

Insulin injection is a lifelong therapy in patients with T1D and insulin-requiring T2D. At the outset, all patients commencing insulin must be counselled about the rotation of insulin injection sites, as frequent injection into a single site can lead to significant hypertrophy of fat tissue – so-called lipohypertrophy. This in turn can lead to erratic absorption of insulin and sometimes erratic hypoglycaemic episodes. Avoidance of injection into lipohypertrophic tissue can help improve glycaemic control.

Easily Confused

1. Other causes of polyuria and polydipsia, and key features

Other causes of polyuria and polydipsia	Key features
■ Diabetes insipidus	■ Normal glucose, lack of production or response to vasopressin; check urine and serum osmolality
■ Hypercalcaemia	■ Normal glucose, high calcium – check parathyroid hormone, and if low, consider malignancy
■ Chronic kidney disease	■ Normal glucose, high urea/creatinine
■ Psychogenic polydipsia	■ Normal glucose, psychiatric history

2. Diabetic peripheral neuropathy and other causes of neuropathy

Diabetic peripheral neuropathy	Other causes of neuropathy
■ Loss of fine touch, vibration, ankle jerks ■ May have burning, tingling, shooting pain ■ Is likely to improve with improved glucose control	■ Consider B_{12} deficiency, especially in patients on metformin ■ Consider alcohol excess, especially in patients with liver or pancreatic disease

3. Autonomic neuropathy and drug-induced postural hypotension

Autonomic neuropathy	Drug-induced postural hypotension
■ Postural hypotension but may have other symptoms such as erectile dysfunction or diabetic gastroparesis ■ May require drugs to increase blood pressure (e.g. midodrine, fludrocortisone, erythropoietin)	■ Commonly associated with alpha-blockers but all antihypertensives may cause symptomatic postural hypotension ■ May require reduction in antihypertensive therapy

4. Hypoglycaemia and transient ischaemic attack

Hypoglycaemia	Transient ischaemic attack
■ Low glucose leading to transient hemiparesis ■ Usually responds quickly to glucose therapy ■ Insulin or sulfonylurea therapy should be reduced	■ Glucose level normal and does not respond to glucose therapy ■ Cardiovascular risk factors should be screened for and treated

Prescribing Points

1. **Metformin: Start it slowly and titrate, and only stop in significant renal impairment**
   a. Metformin may reduce cardiovascular and microvascular complications of diabetes.
   b. Prescribe at a low dose and titrate slowly – 500 mg once daily after the main meal, titrated at weekly intervals to 1000 mg twice daily.
   c. If side effects occur despite these precautions, a modified release may be useful.
   d. Stop when estimated glomerular filtration rate (eGFR) <30 mL/min due to the risk of accumulation.
   e. Reduce when eGFR <45 mL/min.
   f. Sick day rules – avoid metformin during intercurrent illness due to the risk of a sudden drop in renal function. Restart on recovery.

2. **Doses of oral hypoglycaemics and insulin need to be reduced with declining renal function**
   a. Insulin requirements follow a biphasic course in progressive renal disease – in early stages of diabetic nephropathy, resistance to the effects of insulin predominates and may worsen, leading to a greater requirement for insulin.
   b. As eGFR declines, insulin requirements may diminish significantly – lower doses of insulin or sulphonylureas are needed in patients with eGFR <30 mL/min.

3. **Consider treating low testosterone in diabetic men with erectile dysfunction**
   a. Erectile dysfunction in men with diabetes is common and associated with autonomic neuropathy and vascular disease.
   b. Men with T2D appear to be at higher risk of hypogonadism.
   c. Treating low testosterone in men with diabetes may improve quality of life and reduce complications, although firm evidence is lacking.

4. **Many drugs increase the risk of developing diabetes**
   a. Corticosteroids, beta-blockers and thiazides increase glucose levels.

b. Atypical antipsychotics, such as olanzapine, risperidone and clozapine have been associated with drug-induced diabetes.

c. If possible, such drugs should be avoided in patients with diabetes.

5. **Sodium-glucose transporter-2 inhibitors (SGLT-2i) should be used to protect from cardiovascular and renal disease in people with T2D**

a. The latest NICE guidance suggests that SGLT-2i drugs (gliflozins) should be used more widely in people with T2D.

b. Offer SGLT-2i in people with known cardiovascular disease or albumin creatinine ratio >30 mg/mmol.

c. Consider SGLT-2i in people with QRISK2 score >10% or urine ACR 3–30 mg/mmol.

6. **Beware the risk of certain drugs**

a. SGLT-2i may rarely cause euglycaemic DKA. Check urinary or plasma ketones in any person on these medications who presents with acute nausea, vomiting, abdominal pain or breathlessness, even if their plasma glucose is normal.

b. Glucagon-like peptide-1 analogues have been reported to contribute to DKA as a result of large reductions in insulin dosage due to a reduction in appetite or weight loss. They may also increase the risk of pancreatitis and should probably be avoided in people with a previous history of this condition.

EMERGENCIES IN GENERAL PRACTICE

Keith Hopcroft

Ten Pearls of Wisdom

1. **Correct disposal is more important than a clever diagnosis**

   It's always nice to come up with a specific diagnosis – especially if it's correct. But in urgent care, the priority is that the patient is treated in the right place: at home for community care and monitoring, or in hospital for more significant problems. So, using abdominal pain as an example, concern yourself primarily with whether the issue seems 'surgical': new, acute, often constant, worsening, in a patient who may be unable to straighten up or walk, is unwell, and may have features of peritonism and systemic upset. Similarly, know when a child is 'ill'; use the NICE traffic light, sepsis chart, and your own assessment and instinct to guide your actions.

2. **If in doubt, arrange a face-to-face consultation, and always safety-net**

   A quick glance at a patient face-to-face will often tell you more about how sick they are than a long phone conversation or even a video consultation – and your gut response will often be right. The patient will appreciate the personal input, too, as will any potential medicolegal defence. Even then, doubt can remain, so safety-net carefully and be honest about uncertainty. Influenza, for example, is likely in the unwell patient mid-epidemic, but cases of meningitis can have identical early symptoms, so any deterioration requires parents or carers to take urgent action.

3. **Know when to worry about the acute painful red eye**

   This is a common emergency presentation and a knowledge of a few key red flags can help you decide whether the patient needs urgent referral. Chief among these are unilaterality and, particularly, loss of visual acuity (which should be formally checked). Other significant features include pain rather than soreness/grittiness, photophobia, ciliary blush and pupillary abnormalities. Remember to stain with fluorescein if the diagnosis isn't clear and have a very low threshold for referring contact-lens wearers.

DOI: 10.1201/9781003304586-9

59

4. Remember to consider both cause and effect

In some acute presentations, there are two aspects to consider: What has caused the presenting problem, and what might be the resulting effects? So, in the elderly with a fall, you'd need to both explore the various aetiological factors and exclude significant injury. And in a vomiting diabetic, you'd need to consider the extensive differential for vomiting and the possible sequelae of dehydration and deranged blood sugars. If either side of the equation rings alarm bells or is not manageable in the community, admit.

5. Vague or apparently minor symptoms presenting urgently may have a serious cause

In routine surgeries, we can be relatively relaxed about non-specific symptoms with a long history. But such symptoms are uncommonly presented in the urgent context – and if they are genuinely acute, especially in a rare attender, think carefully. That sudden onset of dizziness could be the result of a gastrointestinal haemorrhage or a silent myocardial infarct. Similarly, apparently minor symptoms can herald major pathology – a cerebrovascular accident (CVA) can present with sudden onset of deafness or vertigo, and abrupt limb pain could be acute onset ischaemia.

6. In emergency care, organisation and proactivity are as important as clinical acumen

Get organised and think ahead. You may need to reorder your work according to administrative and clinical needs. For example, if you are lucky enough to have an acute visiting service, scan your triage list for those likely to need a visit so you can arrange this well before the local 'cut-off'. And from a clinical perspective, don't rely on those booking your list to necessarily have the knowledge to order appointments according to medical priority: spotting an appointment for 'painful testicle' in a child nominally booked in for a call later in the day should prompt immediate action. And having an 'urgent care' database on hand will improve your efficiency; this means up-to-date numbers for the acute medical unit, mental health crisis service, frailty team and so on, and easy access to essentials such as sepsis score charts.

7. Don't forget a few key direct enquiries

What the patient or parent volunteers in terms of symptoms and background, together with a brief history and – assuming you have access – the patient's record, will usually provide enough detail for safe and efficient triage. Sometimes, though, essential information might not be forthcoming unless specifically solicited. In an unexplained fever in an adult, for example, a history of travel (think malaria) and questions about occupation (consider Weil's disease) might provide a key clue to the diagnosis. And don't automatically rely on the records for the medication history: it may not be immediately apparent that treatment has recently been supplied or modified elsewhere. This might include significant medication such as immunosuppressants supplied by the hospital, so make a direct enquiry.

8. The combination of crying and lethargy in a baby is worrying

'The crying baby' is a common acute presentation with a huge range of differentials. Specific diagnoses can be difficult as there may be little other information to go on, and there may be few clues on examination, although standard observations like temperature, pulse, respiratory rate, CRT and so on from the familiar sepsis screen can be helpful. In a baby, the combination of abnormal or inconsolable crying with out-of-character drowsiness should be taken very seriously as, regardless of other features, it can herald a serious disease such as meningitis.

9. Do some of your basic observations surreptitiously when dealing with young children

Urgent paediatric assessment is fraught with difficulties. The history is, by default, second hand (in young children at least) and so in assessing whether or not a child is 'ill', the examination assumes disproportionate significance. This is fine in a quiet, cooperative child but nigh on impossible in a screaming, fractious toddler. Assessment can begin in the waiting room. Consider ditching the Tannoy system for children; retrieving the parent and child from the waiting room will tell you a lot about the clinical condition. A child flopped onto their mum's chest is going to concern you more rather than one charging around the waiting room eating crisps. Once in the consulting room, your best chance to get a clear idea of respiratory rate and respiratory distress is when the child is quiet, and that is more likely at the beginning of the consultation when the parent is giving the background – and before you rock the boat by approaching the child with equipment in hand. So it makes sense – especially in a case of fever, cough or breathlessness – for the child's top to be casually and gently lifted by the parent while the child is still calm so that you can make your observations while taking the history. In older children who are fearful of the doctor, a minute or so spent gaining their confidence in a friendly way – showing interest in their dinosaur or unicorn pyjamas often works well – pays dividends when you come to examine them. And encourage parents to buy their offspring a toy doctor's kit and even bring it to future appointments. Familiarity breeds calm.

10. Know when to worry about fever – and when not to

A temperature of 38°C or more in a baby of less than 3 months old and of more than 39°C in a baby between 3 and 6 months old represent a red and amber flag, respectively. Outside those ages, and with a few exceptions, temperature alone is of little help in gauging illness severity, beyond indicating some sort of likely infective process. Parents/guardians should be reassured of this fact and told not to 'obsess about' or 'fight' the fever – a natural and harmless response to infection – and instead to focus on other potential red flags such as overall appearance, level of consciousness and breathing.

Obscure or Overlooked Diagnoses

1. Pericarditis

As soon as we hear that a chest pain is sharp, we tend to relax – at least about myocardial ischaemia. Instead, we usually consider whether this represents musculoskeletal pain or, less commonly, pleurisy from pneumonia or a pulmonary embolus. So it's quite easy to forget to include pericarditis in the differential. This causes a sharp sternal pain which can radiate to the left arm, is eased by sitting forward and may be accompanied by a pericardial rub. In theory, the confident GP with a clear diagnosis might manage this in primary care; in practice, most of us will refer to hospital to confirm the diagnosis, establish cause and exclude complications.

2. Pre-eclampsia causing epigastric pain

Pre-eclampsia is probably not the first thing we'd think of in a pregnant woman beyond 20 weeks gestation with epigastric or right subcostal pain. But it's worth bearing in mind as a possible cause. It results from hepatic congestion and may be accompanied by other pre-eclamptic symptoms such as headache or visual disturbance. So remember to assess for oedema and proteinuria, and check blood pressure in these women – and transfer them immediately to hospital if pre-eclampsia is suspected.

3. Kawasaki disease

Feverish children are a staple of GP emergency duty. Such cases often present with other symptoms such as rash, red eyes and cervical lymphadenopathy, and are usually viral. So it's understandable that the diagnosis of Kawasaki disease is easily missed. The clue is the prolonged fever – 5 days or more – usually in an unwell child younger than 5 years old. A textbook case will have accompanying symptoms of cervical lymphadenopathy, non-purulent conjunctivitis, red cracked lips or tongue, a rash, and reddened and/or swollen extremities, which may peel later in the illness. Note: Some of these features might have resolved by the time of presentation. Prompt referral and treatment can prevent complications such as coronary arteritis and aneurysms.

4. Inhaled foreign body in a child

This is another urgent rarity so easily overlooked because our senses are dulled by the ubiquity of the presenting symptom – in this case, cough. A high index of suspicion is needed. The patient is usually a child under the age of 3 and the best pointers are the absence of the usual preceding or accompanying upper respiratory tract infection (as in viral cough), a witnessed episode of choking (though many are unwitnessed) and the dramatically sudden onset of cough. The cough is paroxysmal and may present days or even weeks after the event, and physical examination may be completely normal. If you've seriously considered inhaled foreign body as a diagnosis, then refer urgently.

5. **Intussusception**

    Episodic crying or screaming in an infant typically makes us think about colic or cow's milk protein intolerance. Bear in mind intussusception as a rare cause, particularly in those 1-year-old or less. This will present acutely with a sudden onset of 'colic'. A key pointer is marked pallor during these episodes; in most other scenarios, the baby will be pink or bright red when crying or screaming. These spasms last for a few minutes and happen around every quarter of an hour; the child will probably be vomiting and this may become bile-stained. You might be able to feel a mass in the right upper quadrant. Do not be misled by the absence of 'classical' blood or mucus in the stool – these are late signs.

6. **Temporal arteritis**

    It's relatively rare for a headache to present as an emergency, so think carefully before deciding the patient doesn't need urgent assessment. Subarachnoid haemorrhage and meningitis are unlikely to be underestimated, but other urgent scenarios might be easy to overlook. Brain tumours might become 'acute' either as the patient or carers lose patience with the progressive pain or develop concerns about associated features. But temporal arteritis is probably the one easiest to overlook; consider this in older patients (always over 50 and usually around 70) with a new severe headache. It can present acutely and may be accompanied by scalp tenderness and jaw claudication. Prompt referral and treatment with steroids are essential to prevent the possible ocular complications.

Easily Confused

1. Vasovagal and anaphylaxis

	Vasovagal	**Anaphylaxis**
Skin	Cold, clammy	Normal or reddened
Pulse	Slow	Fast
Carotid	Good volume	Weak
Wheeze	None	May be present
Urticaria	None	May be present
Facial oedema	None	May be present
Breathing	No breathing difficulty	Breathing difficulty
Recovery	Rapid recovery on lying down with no other treatment	Deterioration with no other treatment

2. Pneumothorax and exacerbation of COPD

	Pneumothorax	*Exacerbation of COPD*
Onset	Immediate/sudden	Over a few days
Preceding URTI	No	Likely
Cough	No	Yes
Purulent phlegm	No	Yes
Pain	Likely	Unlikely
Lung findings	Decreased movement on affected side, reduced air entry on affected side, hyperresonance	Widespread wheeze, crepitations, may be widespread reduced air entry

Note: Patients with COPD are at greater risk of pneumothorax, and this can easily be confused with an acute exacerbation.

3. Pneumonia in a child and bronchiolitis

	Pneumonia	*Bronchiolitis*
Age	Any	Usually age <1
Respiratory distress	Likely	Possible
Temp >39°C	Likely	Unlikely
Unwell	Yes	Possible
Chest findings	Focal crepitations	Widespread wheeze and widespread crepitations

4. Faecal impaction with overflow and any other cause of acute diarrhoea

	Faecal impaction with overflow	*Any other cause of acute diarrhoea*
Age	Very young/very old (though children less likely to present acutely)	Any
Preceding constipation	Yes	Unlikely
Incontinence	Yes	Possible
Otherwise unwell	Unlikely	Likely
Rectal examination	Hard stools impacted in rectum	Soft stools

Prescribing Points

1. Know your adrenaline doses

In most scenarios, even urgent ones, you have time to look up doses – perhaps not at leisure but certainly with some quick clicks of a mouse or scrolling on a phone. Anaphylaxis is probably the exception. Such is the level of urgency and the general sense of panic that you may not have that luxury – and therefore adrenaline doses are ones you might well want to keep in your head (see the following table derived from the BNF). Better still, ensure that any building you work in has a laminate of doses within the emergency box/pack where the adrenaline is kept.

Age	Dose
Up to 6 months	100–150 micrograms
Child 6 months–5 years	150 micrograms
Child 6–11 years	300 micrograms
Child 12–17 years	500 micrograms (300 micrograms if child small or pre-pubertal)
Adult	500 micrograms

In each case:
- Use adrenaline 1 in 1000 (1 mg/mL) injection
- Give by intramuscular route
- Repeat dose after 5 minutes if no response
- Further doses can be given every 5 minutes until specialist urgent care is available
- Inject preferably into the anterolateral aspect of the middle third of the thigh

2. **Remember the DAMN drugs**
   It's easy to manage apparently humdrum cases such as gastroenteritis on something approaching autopilot. But it's worth remembering that the patient's medication might require some extra thought. Some drugs – diuretics, ACEIs/A2RBs, metformin and NSAIDs (DAMN) – put patients (especially the elderly or frail) at risk of renal impairment in the event of a potentially dehydrating illness, and, in the same circumstances, metformin can precipitate lactic acidosis. So these drugs – conveniently prompted by the DAMN acronym – should be stopped for the duration of the illness.

3. **Check the medication history**
   Outside of the DAMN scenario, ongoing medication can put a significant twist on certain consultations, even seemingly mundane ones. Hence, patients on immunosuppressive treatment with common infections such as shingles or a chest infection might need very careful handling – and bear in mind that the relevant medication might not appear in the patient's record if it's hospital-provided or recently initiated. Even the humble sore throat needs deeper thought if, for example, the patient is on carbimazole – in which case the drug should be stopped pending an urgent FBC.

4. **Remember to let the receiving team know what you have given**
   In a real emergency, the provision of a letter for the receiving team may be low down your list of priorities. But they must be aware of any treatment you have provided prior to transfer – such as GTN, analgesia and aspirin in a myocardial

infarct, and adrenaline doses in anaphylaxis. If there is no time to write a letter, you can verbally update the ambulance crew or, later, contact the on-take team, or even text the information to the patient or relative to convey to the hospital.

5. **Stock your emergency cupboard**

The emergency drugs you might need will depend on several factors including local arrangements and practice demographics. The CQC website does provide a suggested list of emergency drugs for GP practices which could be used as the basis for ensuring the main areas are covered. It includes:

- Adrenaline for injection
- Antiemetics
- Soluble aspirin
- Benzylpenicillin for injection
- Dexamethasone oral solution or soluble prednisolone
- Diclofenac injection
- Glucagon
- GTN spray
- Buccal midazolam or rectal diazepam
- Opiates for injection
- Salbutamol via nebuliser

ENT

Andrew Bath, John Phillips, Peter Tassone and Stephanie Cooper

Ten Pearls of Wisdom

1. Most patients describing a 'lump in their throat' do not have cancer – even if that's what they fear

Almost half of adults will at some time complain of a 'lump' or odd discomfort in their throat. There is usually no difficulty in swallowing – in fact, swallowing may help to ease this sensation. Often these patients have gastro-oesophageal reflux or nasal symptoms, or work in air-conditioned environments. Many are extremely anxious, especially about throat cancer. Treating any underlying problem is important, but there is no magic cure for this condition. Reassurance is therefore paramount. It may be necessary for some of these patients to be referred to an ENT specialist who can perform a fibre-optic endoscopy and give the 'all clear'.

2. Pain in the ear is not always caused by the ear

Pain around the ear is common. Unless there is discharge from the ear or a hearing loss, it is unlikely that the pain is due to the ear itself. In young children, this can be difficult to determine, but if they are apyrexial, an acute otitis media is unlikely. Referred pain can come from the throat (tonsillitis), the teeth (molars coming through in children) and the muscles around the jaw joint (temporomandibular joint dysfunction). It is therefore important that these areas are examined as well as the ear. Very rarely, this symptom may be caused by cancer of the throat – especially in patients over 45 years old who smoke.

3. Tinnitus can be treated

It is a myth that tinnitus cannot be treated. In fact, tinnitus often naturally improves with time. In the presence of a hearing loss, hearing aids can be very effective at improving the hearing and camouflaging their tinnitus – even after removing the aids. In a minority of cases, tinnitus can be terribly intrusive; however, cognitive behavioural therapy and mindfulness have been shown to offer good alternative treatments. Informing patients that nothing can be done is both incorrect and harmful.

DOI: 10.1201/9781003304586-10

4. When seeing a patient with 'dizziness', establish exactly what they mean

Dizziness is common and can be a very difficult diagnosis to pin down. It is important to recognise the difference between vertigo (hallucination of movement), presyncope (feeling faint), disequilibrium (unsteadiness) and lightheadedness. By allowing the patient to describe their symptoms in their own words, but without using the word 'dizziness', the vast majority of these presentations can be diagnosed by history alone. However, any loss of consciousness requires exclusion of a cardiac or neurological cause – these patients need to be referred as appropriate.

5. Beware of unilateral nasal discharge – it may have a significant cause

Unilateral nasal discharge can occur at any age due to infection; however, when a unilateral mucopurulent nasal discharge occurs in a child, the possibility of a nasal foreign body should be considered, especially if it is foul smelling and there is excoriation around the nostril. In an elderly patient with a unilateral nasal discharge – particularly if it is tinged with blood – a malignancy needs to be excluded as a matter of urgency.

6. Any unexplained lump in the neck of someone aged 45 and over should be regarded as cancer until proven otherwise

Beware of patients aged over 45 presenting with lumps in their necks. They can often be due to infections, which cause cervical lymphadenopathy, or more specific problems such as a thyroglossal or branchial cyst. However, any 'unexplained' lump over 1 cm in diameter in the neck should raise 'alarm bells', especially in patients over 45 years old who smoke. Even if it appears to be a branchial cyst clinically, in patients aged over 45 there is an increased likelihood that this is a cystic metastasis from a malignancy in the throat such as a squamous cell carcinoma of the tonsil.

7. Treat facial palsy with high-dose steroids promptly unless medically contraindicated

A facial weakness typically presents acutely owing to the visual impact that it has on patients. The most common cause in adults is Bell's palsy, which is a diagnosis of exclusion. There is good evidence that giving high-dose systemic steroids within 72 hours will improve the outcome; however, antiviral treatment is still controversial. Poor prognostic factors include a complete palsy, age over 60 and no sign of recovery by 3 weeks.

8. Treatment of medical problems of the nose needs to be long term

Allergic rhinitis and nasal polyps affect over a third of the population. These conditions are often associated with asthma and in a similar fashion need to be managed medically on a long-term basis. Patients that are symptomatic throughout the year with allergic rhinitis, and those with nasal polyps, require a regular topical nasal steroid spray. Often it may be necessary to also prescribe a systemic antihistamine and possibly a leukotriene receptor antagonist, which act in a synergistic fashion to dampen the inflammatory response in the nasal mucosa.

9. Any significant unilateral cochlear symptom requires exclusion of intracranial pathology

Tinnitus and hearing loss affecting both ears are common; however, unilateral symptoms are less common and require further investigation. The underlying concern is that this could be due to a vestibular schwannoma (acoustic neuroma), a rare, benign, slow-growing tumour. The investigation of choice is an MRI scan. There is no need for this to be done as an 'urgent request' unless the patient has other symptoms that dictate this.

10. Don't forget that reflux can be the cause of various ENT symptoms

Gastro-oesophageal reflux can present in many ways. In some patients, it causes a classic 'burning' sensation in the chest or throat. In others, it may present with symptoms caused by acid irritating the throat, such as hoarseness due to irritation of the larynx and 'globus' symptoms due to irritation of the hypopharynx. Utilising acid-neutralising/acid-reducing medications along with raft-forming agents can work synergistically to treat persistent symptoms.

Obscure or Overlooked Diagnoses

1. **Atypical facial pain**

   Many patients present with 'sinusitis' to their doctor. Often they are describing pain or discomfort over the middle third of their face, and have no other symptoms. If the patient has a high temperature and nasal discharge, a diagnosis of acute sinusitis is likely, especially if the patient has sensitive teeth. However, the majority of patients seen in an ENT clinic have a normal endoscopic examination of their noses. The diagnosis is more likely to be atypical facial pain and is best managed with appropriate analgesics or chronic pain medication such as low-dose amitriptyline.

2. **Malignant otitis externa**

   This is a complication of otitis externa with spread of the infection to the surrounding bone causing osteomyelitis. This typically occurs in elderly diabetic patients or immunocompromised patients. Often the pain is severe and unremitting and disproportionate to the clinical signs. Not uncommonly, cranial nerves can be affected by progression of the inflammation – the most common being facial nerve palsy. Patients should be referred to ENT urgently for aural toilet and appropriate medical and possibly surgical treatment. Before antipseudomonal antibiotics were available, it was often fatal – hence, the term 'malignant'.

3. **Spasmodic dysphonia**

Spasmodic dysphonia is a disorder characterised by vocal fold spasms that most commonly result in a 'strained' and 'strangled' voice. It affects only the speaking voice with shouting, whispering, singing and laughing remaining intact. For this reason, it is often misdiagnosed as a functional voice disorder. There is no cure, but spasms can be relieved by injections of botulinum toxin into the affected laryngeal muscles.

4. **Vestibular migraine**

When a patient with a history of migraine begins to experience vertigo associated with headache or other migraine symptoms, such as visual aura, a diagnosis of vestibular migraine is worth considering. Unlike Meniere's disease, which can cause vertigo lasting from a few minutes to several hours along with hearing loss and pressure sensation over the affected ear, a vertigo attack of vestibular migraine can last for less than 20 minutes or many days. The first line of treatment for vestibular migraine is similar to that of classical migraine, but it is worthwhile asking for the opinion of an ENT doctor in the first instance to exclude competing diagnoses.

5. **Acute sensorineural hearing loss**

This should be viewed as a medical emergency. It is relatively rare and there may be no other symptoms apart from the sudden hearing loss. Examination of the eardrum is normal. Weber's test should show that the sound lateralises to the better-hearing ear and Rinne's test is positive bilaterally. In the rare event of a 'dead' ear (no perceptible hearing), a 'false' Rinne negative may occur due to the sound being heard better due to bone conduction in the 'good' ear. Systemic steroids are usually prescribed and occasionally intratympanic steroids may be given.

6. **Superior semicircular canal dehiscence**

Patients present around the age of 45 with autophony in the affected ear (they can hear their own voice more loudly and will sometimes describe the phenomenon of hearing their own eyeballs move) and tinnitus, which may be associated with loud noises and hyperacusis (sensitivity to sound). This has a gradual onset and is due to a thinning or absence of bone over the superior semicircular canal. If the symptoms are severe, surgical repair may be warranted.

7. **CSF rhinorrhoea**

This may occur from trauma to the head or simply from nose blowing causing damage to an area of congenital weakness around the cribriform plate of the anterior skull base. Patients report a unilateral clear nasal discharge, which can be profuse. This can be made worse by straining or hanging the head down, which is the ideal position to collect some fluid. This fluid should be analysed for beta-2 transferrin, which confirms that this fluid is CSF. Some cases may heal. If symptoms persist, surgical closure utilising an endoscopic approach should be considered.

8. **Atypical mycobacterial infections in children**

This is a relatively rare problem that is seemingly becoming more common, affecting children under the age of 5. The diagnosis is usually made clinically when chronic cervical lymphadenitis with a violet discolouration of the skin persists in spite of broad-spectrum antibiotics. The child is normally systemically very well. Medical treatment with clarithromycin (and sometimes also rifampicin) along with surgical excision may be necessary.

9. **Vasculitis**

Occasionally, the first presentation of vasculitis may be in an ENT clinic. Suspicion is aroused especially when patients do not respond to appropriate treatment for common ENT problems such as nosebleeds, nasal polyps, facial pain, earache and hearing loss, to mention just a few. Sometimes there may also be other, more general, non-specific symptoms such as tiredness. It is important to be aware that vasculitic conditions such as granulomatosis with polyangiitis (formerly known as Wegener's granulomatosis) can present in this way with a wide range of ENT symptoms and for the ENT doctor to have a low threshold for referral to a rheumatologist.

Easily Confused

1. **Vestibular diagnoses**

Disorder	Duration of vertigo	Hearing loss	Tinnitus	Aural fullness
BPPV	Seconds	No	No	No
Recurrent vestibulopathy	Minutes to hours	No	No	No
Meniere's disease	Minutes to hours	Yes	Yes	Yes
Vestibular migraine	Minutes to days	No	No	No
Vestibular neuronitis	Days	No	No	No

2. Peripheral vestibular and psychogenic dizziness

Feature	Peripheral vestibular	Psychogenic dizziness
Duration	Usually seconds, minutes or hours (never a 'flash')	Variable, from a 'flash' to days
Frequency	Except for BPPV, rarely more than once a day	Constant or several times a day
Head movement	Intensifies symptoms	Symptoms usually unaffected
Ataxia during episode	Usually prominent	Insignificant
Effect of hyperventilation	Not like the episode	Often reproduces symptoms accurately

3. Oropharyngeal dysphagia and oesophageal dysphagia

Feature	Oropharyngeal dysphagia	Oesophageal dysphagia
Location of impairment	Lips to cricopharyngeus (upper oesophageal sphincter)	Cricopharyngeus to lower oesophageal sphincter
Common cause	Neuromuscular or anatomical	Abnormal oesophageal motility or obstruction
Timing of problem	Difficult initiation of swallow or dysphagia within a second of swallow	Dysphagia after a few seconds of swallow
Reported symptoms	Coughing, choking	Bolus sticking
Most difficult bolus	Usually fluids	Usually solids

4. Acute otitis media and chronic suppurative otitis media and otitis externa

Feature	Acute otitis media	Chronic suppurative otitis media	Otitis externa
Age	Child	Any age	Adult
Toxic symptoms (pyrexia, feeling unwell)	Yes	No	No
Pain on moving pinna	No	No	Yes
Type of discharge	None until eardrum perforates and then mucopurulent	Mucopurulent or thick discharge	Thick discharge
Hearing loss	Yes	Often	Usually
Appearance of tympanic membrane	Bulging eardrum or perforation with pulsatile discharge	Retraction of eardrum especially in attic region	Normal

Prescribing Points

1. **Reassurance – for most ENT patients this is all that is required**

   Many patients are referred with anxiety-related problems or concerns that they may have something seriously wrong with them. Their symptoms may range from throat discomfort to facial pain to dizziness. A thorough examination and reassurance are often all that is needed. However, some ENT patients may benefit from antidepressants to help alleviate their concerns.

2. **Antibiotics are overprescribed for sore throats and ear infections**

   Sore throats and ear infections are self-limiting infections. Appropriate analgesics are often all that is required in the majority to alleviate the symptoms of patients. Children under 2 years of age are more prone to complications of ear infections and there should be a lower threshold to prescribe antibiotics in this group.

3. **Antibiotic drops in patients who have perforated eardrums**

   Ototoxicity from treating an ear infection with aminoglycoside eardrops in patients with a perforated eardrum is extremely rare. Topical aminoglycosides should be used for no longer than 2 weeks if required. Quinolone topical drops are now often used to treat ear infections in this situation.

4. **Overuse of vestibular sedatives**

   Vestibular sedatives should never be used for more than a few days. There is good evidence that vestibular sedatives prolong recovery by interfering with the natural process of central vestibular compensation. There is also a risk of developing conditions such as Parkinson's disease if taken long term.

5. **Rhinitis medicamentosa**

   This is caused by the overuse of topical OTC nasal decongestants. They are not meant to be used for longer than a week. When used for a prolonged length of time, rebound nasal congestion occurs, causing the patient to increase the dose and frequency, to the point where the patient is left with persistent nasal blockage. Advise the patient to stop taking the medication and use a facial sauna to decongest the nose – this can be especially useful just before going to bed.

FUNCTIONAL SYMPTOMS

Richard Davenport

Ten Pearls of Wisdom

1. 'Functional symptoms' is the best term to use for symptoms not explained by an identifiable cause

It is less likely than other terms – such as medically unexplained, psychogenic and hysterical – to offend or distress patients, and does not have pejorative undertones. Some functional syndromes have acquired specific labels, such as chronic fatigue syndrome or fibromyalgia. Their value is debatable. There are specific definitions of functional neurological disorders (FND) in *ICD-11* and *DSM-5* and terminology in this area remains complicated and evolving. Chronic pain and fatigue are common accompanying symptoms in FND.

2. Reassure patients that functional symptoms are very common

Functional symptoms account for up to 20% of GP consultations and are also very common in secondary care, especially in gynaecology, neurology and gastroenterology. Despite the high prevalence, patients and their families have rarely heard of the term 'functional symptoms', although this is slowly changing. Although functional symptoms are more common in younger women, men and older people are not immune to functional symptoms.

3. Do not diagnose symptoms as functional just because they are bizarre

Beware of leaping to the 'functional' conclusion simply because the presenting symptoms seem weird or are ones that you have never encountered before. Functional symptoms are often stereotypical, following well-recognised patterns – so the more 'odd' a symptom appears, the more likely it is to be disease-based.

4. Keep an open mind

Between 4% and 10% of patients initially diagnosed with functional symptoms eventually end up with an organic explanation (although it's more common

 DOI: 10.1201/9781003304586-11

the other way around and much more difficult to reverse an organic diagnosis). Bear in mind, too, that patients with functional symptoms may also develop identifiable diseases in tandem with their functional issues – in neurology, at least 10% of patients with functional symptoms have an associated disease, and functional symptoms are common in people with established diseases such as MS or myasthenia – so be prepared to reassess symptoms and make both functional and non-functional diagnoses in the same patient.

5. Know the clues

Functional symptoms are often multiple, recurrent, and wax and wane (good days and bad days). Patients may have been investigated in many hospital departments, with unremarkable results leading to extensive medical records. They may have acquired various diagnoses along the way, such as irritable bowel syndrome, functional dyspepsia, asthma and chronic prostatitis. While associated mental health problems are common (around 30%), do not assume that all patients must have psychopathology – a concurrent organic disease is an equally important risk factor. You should, however, actively seek mental health diagnoses (such as depression and anxiety), as these may be treatable.

6. Look for triggers

Although many functional symptoms arise *de novo*, you may be able to uncover certain precipitants. Disease is a common trigger; for instance, an episode of acute vertigo due to acute vestibular failure (labyrinthitis) followed by persisting functional dizziness (persistent perceptual postural dizziness, PPPD) or a faint triggering dissociative (non-epileptic) attacks. Trauma (often relatively minor) and presumed infections are other well-recognised triggers. The term 'post-concussion syndrome' is a misnomer and should be abandoned – patients develop similar symptoms with equal frequency after non-head trauma, and the symptoms are indistinguishable from other functional symptoms not preceded by trauma. Although more research is needed, many people with post-COVID syndrome have very similar symptom phenotypes to other post-viral/post-injury syndromes.

7. Make a confident, positive diagnosis ...

As with most diagnoses, identifying functional symptoms involves pattern recognition. Functional symptoms are typically inconsistent with disease both in nature and variability. Patients may be reluctant to disclose 'odd' symptoms – such as dissociation – or may find them difficult to accurately describe. Avoid placing undue emphasis on previous mental health symptoms, and do not assume your patient is the 'wrong type' (too old/male/nice/sensible) to have functional symptoms. It's important to examine these patients, looking specifically for inconsistent features (e.g. patients may be able to walk backwards much better than walking forwards, or appear to have very weak legs on the couch but be able to stand and walk). These inconsistencies can be useful to demonstrate to patients to help them understand the nature of these symptoms (as opposed to 'catching them out').

8.   ... But use secondary care judiciously

Despite the ubiquity of functional symptoms, secondary care teams are often reluctant to make this diagnosis, preferring either vague labels (functional dyspepsia) or erroneous disease-based diagnoses. GPs should therefore avoid multiple referrals to different specialities (in itself a diagnostic clue), but use secondary care carefully – posing clear and specific questions in any referrals – to help confirm and refine the diagnosis. By definition, investigations into functional symptoms will be unremarkable (other than incidental findings). This does not mean investigations are inappropriate, but they should be carefully chosen and it is important to know when to stop. With modern imaging techniques, it is common to pick up incidental (i.e. irrelevant) findings, which can further complicate matters.

9.   An adequate explanation is essential

Patients with functional symptoms need a confident diagnosis and explanation. Avoid imposing a psychological explanation (e.g. 'stress') – most will be resistant to the idea and it will sour the doctor–patient relationship. Explain what functional means and, to gain your patient's trust – and so improve the chances that the diagnosis is accepted – emphasise that it is not 'all in the head' or the patient is 'putting it on'. Provide reassurance that functional symptoms are common, but do not indicate irreversible damage (which explains normal tests) and thus recovery is possible. Although it can help to reassure about MS or cancer, do not overly focus on telling patients what they do *not* have. If patients throw in new symptoms, amplify existing ones or you hear yourself being repetitive in the consultation, you may well not be 'hearing' whatever it is the patient is trying to tell you.

10.   Know tricks and avoid pitfalls in managing functional symptoms

Management begins with a confident diagnosis and explanation, which may take time and careful liaison with secondary care. Some aspects of functional syndromes may be amenable to drug therapy (e.g. anxiety/low mood or pain), but often patients with functional symptoms end up on too many drugs that have minimal effect; this is especially true of chronic primary pain syndromes. A sympathetic physiotherapist may be helpful for motor syndromes, and in carefully selected patients, psychological interventions may be appropriate. But of most value is the offer of sympathetic and understanding explanations, support, and advice to ease symptoms, improve functioning, and avoid making matters worse. If investigations or referrals are deemed necessary, pre-empt the likelihood of normal results and ensure that expectations aren't raised falsely. Be realistic about what you can achieve – a longer duration of symptoms is a poor prognostic feature.

Obscure or Overlooked Diagnoses

By definition, there are no 'obscure' functional diagnoses, although one might argue that these ubiquitous symptoms are often hidden (or at least invisible to doctors) in plain view! There are multiple labels used for such syndromes and thus much confusion with terminology.

1. **Dissociative attacks/seizures**
   This is the preferred term for symptoms that may otherwise be labelled 'non-epileptic attacks', 'pseudoseizures' and 'psychogenic non-epileptic seizures' (often unfortunately abbreviated to PNES).

2. **Chronic fatigue/fibromyalgia/irritable bowel syndrome**
   The problem with these labels is that they have defined characteristics, yet patients frequently have an 'overspill' of symptoms, which can lead doctors and patients to worry about alternative diagnoses. For example, a patient with long-established IBS develops intermittent sensory symptoms, followed by variable weakness and pain on the left side. This cannot be 'explained' by IBS, thus triggering concerns of a sinister diagnosis such as MS; but in reality, they are more likely different manifestations of functional symptoms. While these may be useful diagnostic labels, remember to be relaxed about inclusion criteria.

3. **Chronic pain**
   Chronic pain without an underlying defined cause is common and causes much misery. It may occur anywhere and can be isolated or associated with functional symptoms. The terminology is confused and confusing; patients often end up (depending on whom they see) with various labels including chronic prostatitis, non-cardiac chest pain, atypical (or idiopathic) facial pain, tension-type headache, piriformis syndrome, hypermobility syndrome, chronic pelvic pain, fibromyalgia, chronic regional pain syndrome, etc. Such labels are unhelpful, encouraging patients (and doctors) to seek the underlying cause which can then be removed. Chronic primary pain is a better term to use.

4. **Persistent postural perceptual dizziness (PPPD)**
   This is a cumbersome term that in itself is obscure, although the symptoms it describes are anything but. It refers to the chronic dizziness/disequilibrium that many complain of, and while it may be triggered by an episode of acute vestibular failure (labyrinthitis), it is not due to persisting vestibular disease.

5. **Debate regarding what is functional and what is not continues**

Perhaps the best example of this is chronic fatigue syndrome, but there are others including postural orthostatic tachycardia syndrome (POTS), hypermobility syndrome, various forms of Ehlers–Danlos syndrome (which is not to suggest that EDS does not exist but such patients commonly describe symptoms indistinguishable from other functional symptoms) and post-concussion syndrome. Post-COVID syndrome (or long COVID) is the most recent addition to this long list, the point being that patients with these various syndromes often describe remarkably similar symptoms for which it is hard to identify a specific underlying disease. More research is needed and the sensitivities are obvious, emphasising the notion that functional symptoms should not be equated with 'stress', 'all in the head', and so on.

Easily Confused

1. Dissociative attacks and epilepsy

Dissociative attacks	Epilepsy
■ Often deny prodromal symptoms, but careful questioning will reveal symptoms of dissociation or panic ■ Often very frequent (multiple attacks/day) ■ Injuries not uncommon, including carpet burn injuries ■ May have preserved awareness during convulsions ■ Waxing and waning, variable, prolonged attacks ■ No true postictal confusion (e.g. recognise family), may be emotional afterwards	■ Either none, or typically recognisable and stereotyped focal onset symptoms ■ Very frequent attacks rare, often tend to cluster ■ Seizure-specific injuries (lateral tongue biting, low back pain/headache, generalised myalgia, shoulder fracture/dislocation) ■ Always unconscious during convulsions ■ Short-lasting, stereotypical episodes ■ Typically disorientated and amnesic after generalised seizures, do not recognise close friends/family

2. Functional hyperventilation and asthma

Functional hyperventilation	Asthma
■ Lack of true reversibility with beta-2 agonists; apparent resistance to treatment ■ Associated features of hyperventilation (dizziness, tingling) ■ Current or previous anxiety or panic attacks ■ Oxygen saturations completely normal even during severe episode	■ Reversibility is the hallmark of asthma; treatment effective ■ Features of hyperventilation... Not present ■ May be no previous or co-existing psychiatric history ■ Oxygen saturations may be reduced during episodes

3. **Functional dizziness (persistent postural perceptual dizziness [PPPD]) and vestibular and central (disease)-based dizziness**

Functional dizziness (persistent postural perceptual dizziness [PPPD])	Vestibular and central (disease)-based dizziness
■ Persistent, pervasive feeling of imbalance/dizziness/ unsteadiness ■ Often exacerbated by visual stimuli (worse in shops/ supermarkets/shopping centres)	■ Usually definable episodic vertigo, and usually possible to categorise as BPPV, acute vestibular failure (labyrinthitis), Meniere's or migrainous ■ Less affected by visual stimuli

Prescribing Points

1. **The role of drugs in functional symptoms is limited**

   Unsurprisingly, given the absence of disease, there are no curative or disease-modifying drugs for functional symptoms, so reliance on drug therapy is doomed to failure. Alternative non-drug approaches including physical and psychologically based therapies are important, but without a clear and coherent explanation of the diagnosis at the outset, lasting success is unlikely. This is particularly apparent in chronic pain, and recent NICE guidelines have recognised the harm of multiple analgesics.

2. **It is difficult to abandon the traditional expectations of doctors and patients that drugs work**

   Modern medicine has fostered the notion of a 'pill for all ill', thus patients often now expect medication – and doctors are often tempted to 'give in', not least because this may be one way to end what can be a difficult consultation. In truth, though, this is no different from the idea of avoiding antibiotics for self-limiting viral infections, as in that scenario, doctors need to appreciate when drugs are not the answer and that explanation is vital, as difficult and time-consuming as this might be.

3. **Polypharmacy is to be avoided**

   Although some patients appear to improve initially with drug therapy (presumably a placebo response), a long-lasting good response is rare, and, as a result, patients often accumulate a long list of medications which have little effect other than harm. An important part of managing patients with long-term functional symptoms includes a critical revaluation and judicious withdrawal of drugs.

4. **Many drugs exacerbate functional symptoms**

   Fatigue, dizziness and dissociation are not only potential adverse effects of many drugs (particular powerful analgesics and those acting centrally) but also common functional symptoms. So, it is easy to see why drugs can exacerbate pre-existing functional symptoms.

5. **Identifying and treating mental health symptoms is appropriate**

   This is one area where drug therapy (with or without psychologically based treatment) may be appropriate and successful, emphasising the importance of identifying relevant psychological factors. The aim of therapy needs careful explanation to avoid the assumption on the patient's part that they are 'mad' and therefore inventing their symptoms.

6. **Don't overlook non-drug therapies**

   Drug therapy for functional symptoms is usually inappropriate and will fail. Physiotherapists (ideally with training in functional syndromes) can be very helpful in managing people with functional motor syndromes. Otherwise, a sympathetic ear and support are more valuable than we think. Above all, GPs have an important role in recognising the 'bigger picture' which is easily missed in secondary care silos, and to a certain extent should protect their patients from the harms that come with overinvestigation and overmanagement at the hands of secondary care teams.

GASTROENTEROLOGY

Stephen J. Middleton and Lisa M. Sharkey

Ten Pearls of Wisdom

1. **Abdominal pain often arises from the abdominal wall – and is easy to confirm**

   Patients referred with abdominal pain often turn out to have pain arising from the abdominal wall (e.g. anterior cutaneous nerve entrapment syndrome), not from within the abdominal cavity. The following simple examination technique can avoid unnecessary investigations: with the patient lying supine, palpate to find the area of tenderness, then ask the patient to slightly raise their head and shoulders off the bed (like halfway to a sit-up). The tender area defined when lying relaxed is now re-examined with the abdominal muscles tense. If the area remains tender, the cause arises in the wall of the abdomen (i.e. is superficial) rather than within the abdominal cavity (as the tensed abdominal muscles would have protected the viscera).

2. **IBS pain rarely wakes people from sleep**

   A common problem in primary care is distinguishing between symptoms likely to be caused by IBS and those which could suggest inflammation or cancer. IBS symptoms of pain or the urge to defecate are unlikely to wake patients from sleep, but patients may report poor sleep, which is actually caused by anxiety or depression. These co-existent mental health conditions may be contributing to the global IBS symptoms. Another more obvious indicator of serious underlying disease is unintentional and significant (>5%) loss of body weight over the preceding few months.

3. **Chronic pain continuing for more than a few hours at the same intensity and in the same location rarely arises from the gastrointestinal tract**

   There are a few important exceptions to this rule, such as pancreatic pain and conditions that have penetrated the wall of the bowel; however, these conditions are usually quite advanced and obvious in other ways by the time they cause this type of pain, so the diagnosis – such as colorectal cancer or penetrating Crohn's disease – should be clear. Chronic pain that radiates to (or from) the back or down

DOI: 10.1201/9781003304586-12

81

the leg/buttock does not usually arise from the hollow viscera and is more likely to be caused by conditions of the musculoskeletal system. Exceptions to this include pancreatic, duodenal ulcer and gallbladder pain, which can all radiate to the back.

4. An isolated moderately elevated ALT in the absence of a clear underlying cause, risk factors or physical signs is likely to be metabolic dysfunction-associated steatotic liver disease (MASLD, formerly known as non-alcoholic fatty liver disease)

On discovering an elevated ALT (normal range <50 IU/L), check the detailed history, looking for risk factors such as high alcohol intake, drug therapy, foreign travel and IV drug use. Also, conduct a physical examination. A liver aetiology screen (Table 12.1) and ultrasound should be performed. If the ALT is modestly elevated (<100 IU/L) in isolation and the aetiology screen is negative, then non-alcoholic fatty liver disease is likely. A FIB-4 score should be calculated to determine the risk of advanced fibrosis (with these patients being referred to hepatology clinic). For low-risk patients, lifestyle modifications or treatments to manage obesity, dyslipidaemia, hypertension and poor diabetic control should be recommended, as appropriate. Patients in the moderate risk group based on FIB-4 should have additional risk stratification with a transient elastography scan (FibroScan®).

5. Some patients with 'constipation' have an evacuatory disorder, in which case escalating laxatives is unlikely to help

Only about half of patients who complain of constipation have slow transit; about 30% have an evacuatory disorder. In this situation, stool is passed along

Table 12.1 Liver aetiology table for patients with non-acute abnormal liver blood tests

	Standard liver aetiology panel	Extended liver aetiology panel
Viral hepatitis	Hepatitis 8 surface antigen and hepatitis C antibody (with follow-on PCR if positive)	Anti-HBc and anti-HBs hepatitis B DNA quantification of hepatitis delta in high-prevalence areas
Iron overload	Ferritin and transferrin saturation	Haemochromatosis gene testing
Autoimmune liver disease (excluding PSC)	Anti-mitochondrial antibody, anti-smooth muscle antibody, antinuclear antibody, serum immunoglobulins	Anti-LKM antibody and coeliac antibodies (consider ANCA in the presence of cholestatic liver blood tests)
Metabolic liver disease		Alpha-1-antitrypsin level; thyroid function tests; caeruloplasmin (age >3 and <40 years) ± urinary copper collection

Source: Newsome PN, et al., Guidelines on the management of abnormal liver blood tests, Gut 2017, doi:10.1136/gutjnl-2017-314924.

Abbreviations: ANCA, antineutrophil cytoplasmic antibodies; LKM, liver kidney microsome; PCR, polymerase chain reaction; PSC, primary sclerosing cholangitis.

the colon to the rectum normally, but the mechanism for evacuating the stool from the rectum is abnormal. A careful history is vital. Patients with slow transit constipation pass hard, dry stools, whereas those with an evacuatory disorder often complain of difficulty evacuating a soft or even loose stool. They may report excessive straining or the need to digitise to remove stool. Many of these patients will be refractory to treatment and receive escalating doses of laxatives that will eventually result in the passage of liquid stool, often with some loss of continence. Diagnosis may require a defecating proctogram and anorectal physiology. Bowel retraining is usually the best mode of treatment, and surgery is reserved for a small number of select cases.

6. Consistent diarrhoea should not be attributed to IBS

Patients with stools that are *consistently* loose are unlikely to have IBS, especially if they do not complain of flatulence. In IBS, the stools usually vary in consistency between hard and loose. There is invariably flatulence, abdominal bloating and discomfort, and the symptoms may be associated with a food trigger and aggravated by stress. Consistent diarrhoea is more likely a sign of serious underlying disease, such as inflammatory bowel disease, infection, microscopic colitis and colonic carcinoma. Bile acid diarrhoea is another relatively common cause (see 'Obscure or overlooked diagnoses'). Other possibilities include bacterial overgrowth of the small intestine and coeliac disease.

7. Bear in mind other possible causes when a patient with altered bowel function returns from a normal 'straight to test' colonoscopy

The actions needed depend on the symptoms. If the patient has chronic watery diarrhoea, review the colonoscopy report to determine if biopsies were taken to exclude microscopic colitis. Occasionally, a patient may need a repeat procedure if this is suspected and no biopsies were taken at the index colonoscopy. Also consider if they could have bile acid diarrhoea, drug-induced symptoms, coeliac disease, small intestinal bacterial overgrowth or constipation with overflow (a clue might be poor bowel preparation noted during the colonoscopy). For a patient referred with new onset constipation and a normal colonoscopy, again consider drug causes initially, but if they fail to respond to first- or second-line laxative treatment, refer to secondary care. Patients with refractory constipation often need multidisciplinary input. Always consider non-intestinal causes of GI symptoms, including systemic diseases or pelvic problems (including ovarian cancer in women).

8. GORD can cause cough, asthma and globus – even when there are no typical GORD symptoms

Gastro-oesophageal reflux disorder (GORD) can cause symptoms other than the usual heartburn/dyspepsia. For example, GORD can provoke asthma, especially in the young. It is also a common cause of chronic cough, usually non-productive, which can persist for many years if the true cause is not identified and treated. Other conditions associated with GORD include dental erosion, halitosis, sinusitis and globus. A detailed history may also reveal evidence of the more traditional GORD symptoms, but in some cases, these are entirely lacking. A trial of proton pump inhibitors (PPIs) can be used but often fails as it may require an extended period of high-dose treatment initially – in combination with alginate-based antacids – to deal with any co-existing bile reflux.

9. **Patients with well-localised upper abdominal pain, increased or decreased by eating, may well have a mucosal abnormality like an ulcer or carcinoma**
Careful consideration should be given to endoscopy in these patients, especially if they are over 50 years old or have associated symptoms such as weight loss or vomiting. Patients with symptoms suggestive of GORD without any alarm symptoms, such as odynophagia or dysphagia, are much less likely to have serious pathology. In patients who complain of ongoing dyspepsia despite a negative endoscopy, remember gallstones as a potential cause.

10. **Serology does not completely exclude coeliac disease – consider duodenal biopsy if the symptoms are highly suggestive**
A coeliac diagnosis is often delayed, as many of the symptoms are similar to those of IBS – and coeliac patients may partly improve with IBS treatment or dietary modification. To add to the confusion, the timing of coeliac symptoms may not correspond to the consumption of gluten; they may be provoked by other foods that are malabsorbed as a result of coeliac disease. Serology for coeliac disease is important in suspected cases but does not completely exclude the diagnosis; 10%–15% of patients with coeliac disease have a negative anti-TTG test. In the face of negative blood tests, where the suspicion of coeliac disease is high (including those who have a first-degree relative with coeliac disease, people with type 1 diabetes or autoimmune thyroid disease, and people with Down's or Turner's syndrome), a duodenal biopsy should be arranged.

Obscure or Overlooked Diagnoses

1. **Oesophageal spasm**
Non-cardiac chest pain is common and in many cases results from an oesophageal spasm. This is often caused by gastro-oesophageal reflux, which may or may not cause typical GORD symptoms, too. Therefore, a trial of PPIs is worthwhile, but failure to respond does not exclude the diagnosis. If the diagnosis is suspected

and PPIs don't help, referral to a specialist may be appropriate, particularly if the symptoms are intrusive.

2. **Obscure dysphagia**

   It is wise to investigate any degree of dysphagia to prevent late diagnosis, as its causes are rarely entirely harmless. Three commonly overlooked causes are:

   a. *Globus*: Patients reporting high dysphagia often have a form of globus characterised by the sensation of something sticking in their throat, high up in the neck. This may be a sign of underlying GORD causing increased tone in the upper oesophageal sphincter. Even when adequate treatment of GORD is administered, it usually takes several weeks before any improvement is noticed.

   b. *Achalasia*: Patients often present late, which can make treatment difficult and less successful. This may be because of the low-grade, insidious onset of the condition, which allows patients to learn methods of managing the symptoms themselves.

   c. *Eosinophilic oesophagitis*: Young patients with dysphagia may have this inflammatory condition of the oesophagus, commonly associated with atopy. Patients often present with intermittent dysphagia or bolus obstruction and if young may not be referred for investigations. Gastroscopy with oesophageal biopsies is required to exclude the diagnosis. It responds very well to steroid aerosols administered via a puffer into the mouth and swallowed (unlicensed but effective), or to an elimination diet.

3. **Bile acid malabsorption-related diarrhoea**

   A cholecystectomy quite commonly leads to consistent bile acid diarrhoea (BAD). This can continue indefinitely unless treated appropriately with resins such as colestyramine. It is important to conduct the usual basic investigations to exclude other causes – particularly as colestyramine can mask symptoms, as it has a constipating effect. There is also an idiopathic form of BAD which can be mistaken for diarrhoea-predominant IBS. Testing for BAD is currently via a SeHCAT (^{75}Selenium homocholic acid taurine) scan, which determines the 7-day retention of labelled bile acids. In the near future, measurement of serum levels of C4 (an intermediary of bile acid synthesis) should be available.

4. **Small intestinal bacterial overgrowth (SIBO)**

   Patients who have this condition may present with abdominal bloating and/or diarrhoea, and are often elderly. The small bowel contains a small number of resident bacterial commensals. If transit through the small intestine is slowed, the number of resident bacteria will increase, leading to mucosal damage and malabsorption. One of the most common causes is the natural decline in the frequency and effectiveness of peristalsis with age. Other causes include jejunal diverticulosis, small bowel strictures and PPI therapy. SIBO should be suspected in someone with symptoms of wind, bloating and diarrhoea, and an underlying predisposition. Glucose hydrogen breath testing has good specificity and reasonable sensitivity in making the diagnosis.

In most cases, the underlying cause cannot be cured, so in the majority, long-term antibiotics are required. These should be given as a rotation between two or three antibiotics to reduce the chances of resistance. Non-absorbable antibiotics such as rifaximin can also be used (though this is off-license use).

5. **Chronic mesenteric ischaemia**

Acute mesenteric ischaemia, due to occlusion of the superior mesenteric artery or vein, is usually acute and severe, with patients profoundly sick. However, chronic ischaemia can be very difficult to diagnose. Atherosclerotic disease of the mesenteric vessels is the most common cause, though the presence of atheroma does not always cause symptoms, because of the collateral network within the abdomen. Patients affected usually have classical cardiovascular risk factors. The symptom of intestinal angina is classically dull, crampy epigastric or central pain, occurring within an hour of eating. Patients will often have lost weight due to the fear of symptoms, which may precipitate investigations for cancer. CT angiography has high sensitivity and specificity for diagnosis.

Easily Confused

1. Incidental gallstones and gallstones-causing symptoms

Incidental gallstones	Gallstones-causing symptoms

■ The finding of gallstones does not always mean that the patient's symptoms are gallstone related.
  ■ If the gallbladder wall is not thickened and there are no features of cholecystitis, the patient's *current* symptoms are unlikely to be due to gallstones.
  ■ However, the patient may still be suffering with biliary colic and should be referred for consideration of cholecystectomy if no other cause of symptoms is found.
	■ The finding of thickening of the gallbladder wall is usually significant, and in the presence of gallstones suggests that cholecystectomy is indicated. When no gallstones are present, a thickened wall may indicate malignancy and the patient should still be referred to secondary care.

2. Food allergy and food intolerance

Food allergy	Food intolerance
■ This is uncommon, usually associated with allergies to other substances and occurs every time the substance (allergen) is consumed. There may be an associated rash and urticaria. There are reliable blood and skin prick tests for this condition.	■ This is common, not associated with allergies and often intermittent. There are no fully reliable tests for this condition and no associated rash.

3. Diverticulosis and diverticulitis

Diverticulosis	Diverticulitis
■ Diverticulosis is the presence of diverticula in the bowel and does not imply that these are causing symptoms or inflammation. This should not be described as diverticular disease.	■ Diverticulitis describes inflammation of the diverticula and can lead to severe symptoms and complications such as colonic perforation. This may be termed diverticular disease.

4. Diarrhoea caused by infection and diarrhoea caused by inflammatory bowel disease

Diarrhoea caused by infection	Diarrhoea caused by inflammatory bowel disease
■ Sudden onset. ■ Diarrhoea is maximal at onset and tails off over a days or weeks. ■ Blood in stools can occur in certain bacterial infections; weight loss often occurs but is short-lived and usually less than 10% of body weight. ■ Faecal calprotectin is elevated initially, but repeat testing after resolution of symptoms will show a lower or normal result.	■ Symptom onset is insidious and builds up to a maximum over days or weeks. ■ Blood in stools is often a feature. ■ Weight loss is more likely in Crohn's disease and can be chronic and progressive until treatment is effective. ■ Faecal calprotectin is elevated.

Prescribing Points

1. **Treatment of GORD with acid blockers**

   PPIs may need to be administered in high doses to control symptoms. It is preferable to start with a high-dose regime and then step down when the symptoms are controlled. Nocturnal acid suppression is augmented by the use of H2 antagonists taken last thing in the evening, along with daytime PPI therapy.

2. **Anal fissures**

   GTN paste for anal fissures is effective but often leads to severe headaches and can cause presyncope and occasionally syncope. Diltiazem 2% paste (unlicensed) is a better alternative – with better compliance – although more expensive.

3. **Personalised IBS treatment**

   IBS is subclassified into diarrhoea-predominant (IBS-D), constipation-predominant (IBS-C) and mixed (IBS-M), and treatment should be directed to the subtype and/or predominant symptom. Effective treatments for abdominal pain and global IBS symptoms include soluble fibre supplementation (starting at

3–4 g per day), antispasmodics and peppermint oil (though the latter may cause GORD symptoms). If loperamide is used to control diarrhoea, start at the lowest dose and slowly uptitrate to avoid side effects. Agents such as ondansetron can also be effective for IBS-D (but this is an unlicensed indication). PEG-based laxatives are the first-line recommendation for IBS-C. When using tricyclic antidepressants or SSRIs, an explanation of IBS as a disorder of gut–brain interaction is essential to facilitate shared decision-making and improve concordance with treatment.

4. **Development of GORD symptoms after eradication of *Helicobacter pylori***
   During infection with *H. pylori*, the gastric mucosa is inflamed and dysfunctional such that, in many cases, gastric acid production is reduced, masking associated GORD. However, eradication of *H. pylori* leads to the restoration of healthy, fully functional gastric mucosa and therefore normal acid production. As a result, patients may develop GORD symptoms from acid reflux. This can cause confusion, as it may seem that the *H. pylori* treatment has not been a success.

GENERAL PRACTICE

Keith Hopcroft

Twenty Pearls of Wisdom

1. **Patients want to know what isn't wrong as much as they want to know what is**

   From day one at medical school, we're taught that medically assessing the patient is all about refining the various pathological possibilities to enable us to clinch the diagnosis. In general practice, this is wrong – up to 75% of primary care presentations evade a specific diagnosis, even after investigation. But that doesn't matter. Because, more often than not, the patient is more interested in knowing what isn't wrong than what is. There is some evidence for this, with a key factor in patients attending for dyspepsia being a fear of cancer. And every day, GPs see patients who, for example, are less interested in knowing that they have tension headaches than in being reassured that they don't have a brain tumour. So there remains value in the cliché, 'I don't know what it is, but I know it isn't serious'.

2. **Most patients presenting with tiredness as a sole symptom do not have a demonstrable physical illness**

   I firmly believe this to be true. Tiredness mentioned in the context of other symptoms – especially weight loss – is a different matter and may have many serious causes. With other suggestive features, patients may have specific syndromes such as chronic fatigue or sleep apnoea (though the latter tends to present with sleepiness rather than tiredness). And depression may well be described as 'tiredness'. But as a presenting complaint, without other symptoms, tiredness rarely turns out to be anything significant. And if the inevitable blood screen does reveal, say, a borderline thyroid or low ferritin, correction of the abnormality rarely leads to any improvement.

3. **Always ask, 'Why are you here, and why now?'**

   Trainees are used to seeing patients in hospital, where the agenda – a need for admission or the clarification of a diagnosis – has often been set by a doctor in A&E or primary care. In contrast, patients attending the GP have – by and large – made their own decision to attend. Satisfactorily resolving their issue,

DOI: 10.1201/9781003304586-13

therefore, requires the GP to drill down into what, exactly, made them take the trouble to book an appointment. Ignore this and you'll overlook astonishing agendas, such as an elderly man I once saw who only decided to have his long-term stiff neck checked out (diagnosis: cervical spondylosis) because his grandson had just been to hospital with meningitis (having presented, yes, with neck stiffness).

4. Children pointing to their umbilicus rarely have a serious cause for their abdominal pain

I've heard many GPs repeat this gem and it has certainly never let me down. It seems to hold true for both acute and chronic bellyache. Perhaps the explanation is that psychogenic pain is truly central or that the young malingerer assumes the belly button must be the focus of all convincing pathology. It follows that the farther the pain appears to be from the umbilicus, the greater the chance of organic pathology and the more the GP should 'beware'.

5. The patient who self-diagnoses is usually wrong

This gem is possibly becoming less valid as patients nowadays have easier access to higher-quality self-diagnostic information. And there is evidence of an important and counterintuitive exception – in that patients who believe their chest pain to be cardiac have a higher chance of that being the case. Nonetheless, my experience with patients worried about diabetes, anaemia, hypothyroidism and so on is that they are invariably wrong. So, too with depression – 'I think I'm depressed' usually turns out to be normal life stress. And also with dementia – most patients self-diagnosing dementia are stressed or depressed, whereas patients with genuine dementia are unaware of or unwilling to accept their problem, and so tend to be presented by concerned relatives.

6. Beware the rare attender

Rare attendance is, for me, the greatest red flag of all. It can also drive a coach and horses through other gems. For example, I would be extremely concerned about a rare attender who presents with, say, tiredness, even in the absence of other symptoms. Conversely, the odds of a very frequent attender having serious pathology is low, especially with 'routine' symptoms such as tiredness, dizziness or cough. Then again, in these patients, so too are the odds of significant illness, at some point, being missed.

7. Think Parkinson's disease in the elderly

I say this because of the number of times I've missed this diagnosis. There are three reasons for this. First, it is a great mimic of depression, dementia, hypothyroidism and so on. Second, it tends not to present with textbook symptoms of, say, a pill-rolling tremor, but with non-specific features such as stiffness, slowing up, falls and 'he's just not himself, doctor'. And, third, continuity of care can, for once, prove counter-productive, as overfamiliarity with the patient means that signs obvious to others might be perceived by the usual GP as 'normal for him'.

8. Check the records to confirm symptom duration

It is extraordinary how often patients will claim that their headaches, for example, are a completely new problem, but scrutiny of their records reveals that these symptoms have been going on for years. The 'search' facility on GP record software makes fact-checking very easy. The explanation for these inaccurate histories may be patients genuinely forgetting the true duration of their symptoms, or it might be a deliberate attempt to get the doctor to take a fresh look at their problem. Whatever, knowing that their symptoms have actually been present for years rather than weeks is both reassuring and informative.

9. If you find you are repeating yourself to a patient, something may have gone wrong with the consultation

Some repetition is, of course, appropriate, such as when you are summarising or want to emphasise something. But sometimes we find ourselves repeating – or even re-repeating – our diagnosis or management plan, especially as a way of trying to end the consultation. These repetitions can sound increasingly forced or even desperate. This may well indicate that you have taken a wrong turn in your consultation navigation. It may be that the patient is not convinced by your explanation, is too anxious to take it in, or that you've not covered a particular concern. Best to back-pedal, acknowledge the problem and explore why the patient doesn't seem aligned with your way of thinking. And try – if not start – again.

10. If the patient has received three unplanned visits in quick succession, admit

I've heard this said by many GPs and, while apparently arbitrary, it makes perfect sense on two levels. First, three visits for the same problem – outside of sensible planned or palliative care, of course – implies either diagnostic uncertainty, a rapidly deteriorating situation, or overwhelming patient or family anxiety. And, second, this level of workload is difficult to sustain. Either way, admission for assessment and stabilisation is a sensible and safe path to take.

11. Proactively explain why an X-ray or scan isn't necessary

It took me a while to figure out why my careful assessment and sensible management plan in patients with – to take two common examples – tension headaches or knee arthritis seemed to leave them dissatisfied. The explanation was the high expectation of investigations – specifically, to take these examples, a brain scan or an X-ray. Failure to arrange these tests was interpreted as the doctor not taking the problem seriously. So now I tend to assume that's part of the agenda and take time to proactively explain why these investigations are usually unnecessary.

12. The patient who makes you depressed is probably depressed

This is another 'old chestnut', but that doesn't make it any less true. Patients with genuine depression rarely present with that – instead, they complain of tiredness, dizziness, malaise and so on. Or they attend repeatedly, with vague symptoms which are difficult to pin down and therefore impossible to treat. As a result, they can elicit a sense of dejection in the GP – and reflecting that back may be the first step in uncovering the true diagnosis and making some real progress.

13. Ask the patient, 'Is there anything else?'

Given the constraints of the 10-minute appointment, inviting the patient to add another problem to whatever they've already presented with sounds perverse. Yet, paradoxically, it can save time. That's because the patient's opening gambit may be a 'passport symptom' rather than the main agenda. If this is pursued immediately, the unwary GP can waste 90% of the consultation dealing with the irrelevant, with the patient only revealing the real issue right at the end, prefaced by the dreaded, 'While I'm here …' So if you suspect there's more the patient wishes to discuss, it helps pace the consultation to establish this from the outset.

14. If the patient hasn't taken any analgesia for a painful condition, then it's unlikely to be serious

This probably applies regardless of the precise condition but is most commonly encountered with back pain. The superficial explanation for this gem is that, if the patient hasn't taken any painkillers, then it can't be that painful – and that, in turn, reduces the likelihood of significant pathology. There's probably more to it than that, though. A lack of self-treatment suggests the pain may not be the real issue. So there's likely to be some other agenda – an underlying worry, sickness certification and so on – which, again, means that red flags are unlikely to be raised.

15. If the eGFR is low in a man, put a hand on his abdomen

Purely clinical gems are hard to come by in general practice, so I'm happy to include this one. For GPs, the discovery of various levels of CKD is a common finding via 'routine' blood testing. So much so that it's easy to slip into 'autodoc' and ignore potential remediable causes – not least because there aren't many. One such, especially in men, is chronic outflow obstruction. I have seen a number of men whose CKD was the result of chronic urinary obstruction secondary to prostatic hypertrophy, revealed by the palpation of a huge bladder. Not all had urinary symptoms, and some had significant improvement in renal function when the underlying issue was treated.

16. Set realistic goals

Have you ever wondered what you're trying to achieve when dealing with patients with, say, fibromyalgia? It certainly can be a frustrating condition to treat, for doctors and patients alike. There are many well-recognised reasons for this, but one worth considering is the fact that no treatment is likely to resolve all symptoms. Making this explicit from the outset, and therefore setting a goal of, say, a 50% reduction in symptoms, means that the management becomes more realistic and therefore more likely to 'succeed'. And this method of avoiding banging your head against a brick wall can be applied to many other chronic pain syndromes.

17. Warn patients about the likely duration of symptoms

Many patients – and some doctors – are surprised at how slowly minor health issues resolve. Examples include the common cold, a simple cough and a back strain, which may take 2, 3 or 8 weeks, respectively, to settle down. Quoting timeframes such as these can reassure patients that the duration of their symptoms is normal and so – hopefully – reduce unnecessary reattendance.

18. A petechial rash found only above the nipple line in an otherwise well child is very unlikely to be serious

A petechial rash in a child is always likely to ring alarm bells. The more acute the onset and the more unwell the child, the louder those alarm bells should be. The usual worry is meningococcal septicaemia, but in less 'hot' cases, there is still the worry of a serious haematological disorder. One situation where the GP can probably relax is when, in an otherwise reasonably well child, the petechial rash is restricted to the distribution of the superior vena cava – in other words, only found above the nipple line. This is rarely caused by a serious disease and instead typically results from suddenly raised intravascular pressure, as after a vigorous cough or vomiting.

19. Sometimes, only a face-to-face will do

The COVID-19 pandemic taught us something we already knew: that many consultations can effectively be dealt with remotely to the satisfaction of both GP and patient. But after 'remote' temporarily became the default, we did, eventually, find the pendulum swinging back the other way. Even if patients didn't necessarily need F2F assessment, many appreciated it and, as a result, were more prepared to accept our diagnoses and advice. In truth, we'd probably underestimated the therapeutic value of human contact. Hopefully, we now have the balance right, mixing remote convenience for some with F2F reassurance for others – so that the recurrent complaint that 'no one's even seen me!' is a thing of the past.

20. Always listen to the whisper in your ear

This is another gem I'd heard from wise senior GPs who would tell me tales of unexplained hunches – sometimes waking them in the middle of the night – which turned out to be correct. I was always a bit sceptical of this. Until, that is, the whisper in my ear was loud enough to send me back to a febrile, pale child I had just visited and was literally about to drive away from. It told me that I had done a perfunctory assessment and that the child might have been more ill than I thought. I went back to the house, reassessed the child and decided he was indeed sicker than I'd imagined and required admission. Two hours later, he was in ITU with epiglottitis. This story is true and was quite probably the germ of the idea that became this book.

Obscure and Overlooked Diagnoses

This is an idiosyncratic list comprising diagnoses you do occasionally see in general practice but which aren't always recognised for what they are –

1. Migrainous vertigo

A specific diagnosis for recurrent vertigo can remain elusive. But a relatively common – and often overlooked – diagnosis is migraine. The vertigo can precede, accompany or follow a headache. It is this association and the recurring nature of the problem which gives the diagnosis.

2. Carbon monoxide poisoning

This is notoriously difficult to diagnose, as the symptoms – headache, nausea, and concentration and memory lapses – are vague and common, and the diagnosis is simply not something we tend to think of. Clues include more than one household member being affected without there being an obvious viral aetiology and symptoms improving while out of the house. For obvious reasons, winter is the time it's most likely to be encountered. Refer to hospital for a definitive diagnosis if suspected.

3. Keratosis pilaris

Keratosis pilaris is extraordinarily common in children and adolescents and yet often misdiagnosed or unrecognised. This condition causes small discrete papules on the outer upper arms and thighs, giving the skin a coarse, sandpaper-like feel. Moisturisers may help, but the condition tends to improve anyway over the years.

4. **Burning legs syndrome**

   Also known as 'burning feet syndrome', burning legs syndrome is common, though only rarely given this official 'label'. It causes unpleasant burning sensations in the legs and feet, mainly in those over 50 and especially at night. A neuropathy-type blood screen is recommended, but most cases are idiopathic. Anti-neuropathy-type treatments may help.

5. **Burning mouth syndrome**

   This is apparently a dentist's heartsink symptom. It's common, the cause is unknown and it's difficult to treat. The usual sore-mouth suspects – such as iron deficiency – need excluding and there must be no visible lesions. It's especially common in perimenopausal women, may be a form of neuropathy, has associations with depression and anxiety (though whether cause or effect is not clear) and, as for burning legs, may respond to anti-neuropathy-type treatments.

6. **Chondrodermatitis**

   This is a small, tender, possibly ulcerated papule on the ear (typically the helix in men and the anti-helix in women). The tenderness may disturb sleep. Treatment involves relieving pressure from the nodule – such as sleeping on the other side – and a range of curative options including steroid injection, cryotherapy and surgery.

7. **Proctalgia fugax**

   This is a severe, short-lived cramping pain in the rectum typically waking the patient at night. The episodes are infrequent, though may cluster, and, in between, there are no gastrointestinal symptoms at all (unless there is co-existing IBS, with which it may be associated). It's thought to result from spasm of the anal sphincter. Treatment isn't usually required – beyond reassurance – though inhaled salbutamol can ease an attack.

8. **Levator ani syndrome**

   This is thought to be caused by spasm of the pelvic floor muscles but, being a less clear-cut symptom with a wider differential than proctalgia fugax, is harder to diagnose in primary care. The typical symptoms are an ache or pressure high in the rectum, usually in a woman, which is constant or regular, in the absence of an obvious cause. The diagnosis is likely to be made in secondary care after referral to exclude other possibilities.

9. **Balanitis xerotica obliterans**

   This is lichen sclerosis of the penis and most commonly manifests in primary care as a sore, itchy, whitish, thickened and scarring foreskin, which may be increasingly difficult to retract. It is almost invariably misdiagnosed initially as candidal balanitis, so consider this in men returning for more of their 'thrush cream'. Potent steroid creams may solve the problem, otherwise, circumcision is needed.

10. **Orgasm headache**

    As the name suggests, this is a headache occurring at the point of orgasm. It can be severe and dramatic, and if only experienced once or twice, then a subarachnoid – or its sentinel bleed – would need excluding. Recurrent orgasm headache at least indicates a harmless cause. It may be a form of migraine, and beta blockers, triptans or indomethacin can be used pre-emptively.

11. **Tietze's disease**

This is a costochondritis usually affecting the second or third rib, resulting in a palpable swelling. The discomfort – and especially the swelling – can last weeks or longer.

12. **Myokymia**

An utterly harmless fasciculation of muscles around the eye. It is very common in the general population but only rarely presented to the GP – and then usually in a patient who is concerned that it is a harbinger of neurological doom. Reassurance is all that is required.

13. **Middle ear myoclonus**

This is sometimes also known as myoclonus of the intratympanic muscles. It results in a characteristic form of tinnitus described as paroxysms of fluttering, flickering or clicking within the ear. Palatal myoclonus can cause similar symptoms. It is described as rare, but it may well be that it is simply not recognised. Treatment is difficult and will require referral if simple reassurance is inadequate.

14. **Meralgia paraesthetica**

This is a nerve entrapment of the lateral cutaneous nerve of the thigh. This results in unpleasant persistent or intermittent sensations – such as burning, tingling or itching – in a distinct area on the anterolateral aspect of the thigh. The cause is usually unclear though it may be associated with obesity. It may resolve spontaneously and weight loss and avoiding carrying objects (phones, wallets and so on) in front pockets may help.

Easily Confused

1. Influenza and meningitis

Influenza	Meningitis
During flu season	Any time but winter commonest
Starts to improve after a few days unless complications	Progressive deterioration
A cough invariably develops	Cough unlikely
No rash	May be non-blanching petechial rash

Note: It is notoriously difficult to distinguish and patients erroneously believe we have some magical power to do so. At the very least, explain that deterioration needs urgent reassessment and if in real doubt, admit.

2. Cellulitis and varicose eczema

Cellulitis	Varicose eczema
Usually unilateral	May be bilateral or unilateral
Painful and tender rather than itchy	Itchy rather than painful and tender
May be systemic upset	No systemic upset
No crusting	Crusting

Note: Just to make it more difficult, varicose eczema can become secondarily infected, i.e. develop into cellulitis, so both diagnoses might co-exist.

3. Gout and septic arthritis

Gout	Septic arthritis
Previous episodes	No previous episodes
Minor, or no, systemic upset	Systemic upset
Big toe most likely	Any joint
Painful to move joint	Almost impossible to move joint

4. Conjunctivitis and other significant red eye

Conjunctivitis	Other significant red eye
Bilateral (though may start as unilateral)	Unilateral
Discomfort, itchiness or grittiness rather than pain	Painful
No significant photophobia	May be marked photophobia
Vision normal (other than some blurring via discharge)	Vision reduced
Pupils normal	Pupil may be abnormal
Discharge tends to be sticky	Any discharge tends to be watery
Ciliary blush absent	Ciliary blush present
Redness affecting bulbar and palpebral conjunctiva	Redness does not affect palpebral conjunctiva

5. Polymyalgia rheumatica and osteoarthritis

Polymyalgia rheumatica	Osteoarthritis
Age over 50 (and usually rather older)	Can affect younger age groups
Pain and stiffness worse first thing in the morning	May be worse after resting, but early morning symptoms less obvious
ESR/CRP usually elevated	ESR/CRP normal
Dramatic response to prednisolone	Little or no response to prednisolone

Prescribing Points

1. **Before you escalate treatment, check the computerised drug history**
   Patients may claim perfect concordance with, say, their asthma or antihypertensive medication, but their script issue history may tell a very different story.

2. **Review repeats for prochlorperazine**
   This drug has traditionally been viewed as a panacea for dizziness. It's only effective in true vertigo – and, then, only in certain types – and, ironically, can cause dizziness as a side effect.

3. **Write the drug indication on the repeat template**
   This acts as a useful reminder for the GP, especially in those drugs with multiple indications, and, if appearing on the prescription, reinforces for the patient the purpose of the drug.

4. **Whenever you see a strange rash, consider a drug reaction (including one to OTC medication)**
   Also, bear in mind that an allergy to antibiotics can take up to two weeks from the first dose to appear.

5. **Some patients seem to be intolerant of just about every medication you try**
   It's not clear whether this is a physical or psychological issue, but it certainly happens. In this case, rather than try the umpteenth antihypertensive, it might be worth clarifying whether the patient wants to continue to pursue the problem.

6. **Explain to patients about multi-indication drugs**
   Otherwise, many patients will be put off; for example, amitriptyline for their sciatic pain when they have read that it's a tricyclic antidepressant.

GENERAL SURGERY

N.F.W. Redwood

Ten Pearls of Wisdom

1. **With peripheral vascular disease (PVD), remember: life before limb before length**
   a. *Life*: Patients with claudication are at increased risk of myocardial infarction, cerebrovascular accident and death. Once PVD is diagnosed, secondary cardiovascular prevention is required.
   b. *Limb*: Those at risk of limb loss have absent pulses with either rest pain or tissue loss. Rest pain is felt in the distal foot or toes (not the calf), initially occurs at night, and ultimately becomes constant. Tissue loss includes necrosis, gangrene or ulcers. Both these groups need urgent referral to the vascular clinic.
   c. *Length*: There is no agreed 'walking distance' at which patients should be referred. Consider in terms of social requirements (jobs and hobbies). Check, too, if walking is also limited by cardiorespiratory or neurological disease, in which case, no benefit will be gained by treating the leg. Note that if a patient has claudication, rest pain or tissue loss, the decision to refer is based on the clinical situation, not the ankle–brachial pressure index (ABPI).

2. **In a patient with varicose veins, leg pain may well have some other cause**
   Symptoms in the legs are common, and so are varicose veins. A false connection is often made between the two. Genuine varicose vein discomfort is felt over the veins, or the leg feels generally heavy or aches. The symptoms deteriorate as the day goes on, and are improved by walking or wearing compression hosiery. Veins do not cause a limp, pain at rest or pain immediately on standing. Localisation of the symptoms is important, as musculoskeletal disorders of the knee, ankle or foot are often overlooked once varicose veins are seen. Patients with skin changes (ulceration or lipodermatosclerosis), recurrent thrombophlebitis or bleeding need referring. Small asymptomatic veins should be left alone. Patients with large symptomatic

DOI: 10.1201/9781003304586-14

veins should be referred for discussion rather than the expectation that they will be offered surgery.

3. Bypass grafts need urgent referral for any new problems

Any patient with an arterial bypass graft who suffers recurrent symptoms, however minor, needs immediate discussion with the vascular team. The return or worsening of claudication might suggest the graft has a stenosis that could be treated by angioplasty. If the foot feels cold, numb or develops rest pain, the graft may have occluded. The sooner intervention takes place, the more likely the outcome will be successful. Often, patients present late despite being told to attend urgently. Have a very low threshold for prompt referral.

4. Breast pain alone is rarely a sign of sinister pathology

This may be considered almost 'normal'. If neither patient nor GP can feel a lump, and there are no changes suggestive of inflammatory breast cancer (erythema, peau d'orange, skin thickening) or an abscess (tender red lump in women who are usually either breastfeeding or are smokers), women with either unilateral or bilateral breast pain can be reassured. NSAIDs are the only treatment shown to help symptoms, which usually resolve spontaneously. If the pain persists for 3 months, then consider referral – but not under the cancer pathway.

5. Any sort of nipple discharge that only appears on squeezing is not pathological

Nipple discharge should only be referred if spontaneous; urgently if over 50 or bloodstained. Any sort of discharge that only appears on squeezing is not pathological and the patient should simply be advised not to squeeze. Small amounts of creamy/milky discharge in women who have had children are likely to be physiological. In other groups with bilateral milky discharge, consider endocrine causes such as pituitary tumours and review the medication (prescribed, alternative and illegal). If in doubt, refer to the endocrine clinic.

6. Not all blue or cold feet need referral

Patients confined to a wheelchair because of strokes, multiple sclerosis, spinal injury, poliomyelitis or other neurological conditions often have very cold feet. In addition, the feet will go a deep blue on dependence. This reflects dysfunction in vasomotor control because of the underlying neurology and not peripheral vascular disease. The colour returns once the leg is elevated, and foot pulses are usually palpable. In the absence of other symptoms or tissue loss, they do not need referral. Reassurance is all that is required.

7. Not all hernias need referral

Not all umbilical or paraumbilical hernias need referral. If they are easily reduced and asymptomatic, patients can be given the option of leaving them alone, though there is a small, unpredictable risk of strangulation. Similarly, small asymptomatic, easily reducible inguinal hernias, especially in the frail or elderly, can be left after discussion. Parastomal hernias do not necessarily need referral, either. Treatment is only offered for those with pain or symptoms of obstruction, or whose stoma appliance will not stay in place. Femoral hernias, on the other hand, need referring because there is a high risk of strangulation. Don't forget that symptomatic hernias in the extremely unfit might have a local anaesthetic option for repair.

8. Divarication of the recti is not a hernia

This is a common finding. It is due to laxity of the linea alba but does not represent a hernia. It is common after multiple pregnancies. It appears as a smooth uniform swelling in the midline on straining between the two rectus muscles. There is nothing to feel on relaxation, and no discrete lump or palpable defect as would be expected with a hernia. Exercise might be beneficial for small defects. Surgical outcomes are unpredictable. Reassurance is the mainstay of care.

9. Most acute cholecystitis can be managed in the community

Pain in itself is not an indication for admission. Only if it cannot be controlled or is worsening should referral be made. It is very important to examine the abdomen. If the gallbladder is palpable, the tenderness extends beyond the right upper quadrant or there is jaundice, it is sensible to ask for a surgical opinion. If you are able, calculate the NEWS2 score. If the score is 3 or less (and not 3 in any category), it is safe to manage the patient at home. Give good pain relief, prescribe oral antibiotics as per your local guidelines, check the liver function and arrange an ultrasound. If there is any deterioration, a further opinion is advised. Once the blood results and ultrasound are available, refer to surgical outpatients

10. Guarding is important – but it is not a voluntary contraction of the abdominal muscles

If you press suddenly or hard enough on any abdomen, the patient will contract the abdominal muscles. This is not guarding. Guarding is an involuntary contraction of the abdominal muscles due to underlying peritoneal inflammation. The best way to elicit the sign is to examine the abdomen gently with the patient distracted. The examining hand will feel the reflex contraction of the abdominal wall muscles like a patellar reflex. This is an important sign. It is very hard to fake and it will help distinguish between genuine pathology and the anxious patient. Rebound tenderness should not be tested for. There are many false positives and it is a cruel thing to do to a patient with genuine peritoneal inflammation.

Obscure and Overlooked Diagnoses

1. **Carotid artery aneurysms and carotid body tumours**
   True aneurysms in the carotid vessels are very rare but need treatment. The majority of patients presenting with pulsatile neck swelling have easily palpable vessels, either because they are thin or because the vessels are tortuous with age. If in doubt, arrange an ultrasound. A non-pulsatile mass next to the carotid bifurcation may be a carotid body tumour. These need referral to the vascular clinic.

2. **Non-atheromatous claudication**
   Some young patients without peripheral vascular disease give a good history of intermittent claudication. There might be a non-atheromatous cause; possibilities include anatomical variation causing popliteal artery entrapment, persistent sciatic artery with congenital absence of femoral vessels or medial cystic disease of the popliteal artery.

3. **Obturator hernia**
   This is rare and very difficult to diagnose. Initially, there may only be pain down the medial aspect of the thigh because of irritation of the obturator nerve. There may also be episodes of resolving small bowel obstruction or acute full-blown obstruction.

4. **Calf muscle hernia**
   This results in a lump on the medial aspect of the calf on standing. It is caused by a small defect in the deep fascia allowing muscle to protrude. It can be confused with a varicose vein; key discriminators are that, often, the defect can be felt in the fascia, it cannot be emptied and it has no Doppler signal. No treatment is required.

5. **Lumps on the head**
   Most scalp lumps are benign but beware of lumps near the angle of the orbit, as they may be angular dermoids which connect deeply. Also be cautious about anything that does not completely look or feel like a sebaceous cyst or lipoma, as it might be a malignant deposit with a large blood supply or connect intracranially. Remember that lumps near the angle of the jaw which look like lipomas are parotid in origin until proven otherwise. Most head lumps can be removed safely in primary care, but if there is any doubt, refer.

6. **Sister Mary Joseph nodule**
   This presents as a hard lump at the umbilicus and represents a metastatic deposit from intra-abdominal malignancy. It can be confused with a hernia. However, it is irreducible and much harder than a hernia.

7. **Spigelian hernia**
   This unusual hernia presents as a soft lump lateral to the rectus muscle in the lower half of the abdomen. It feels like a deep lipoma and may

not have a cough impulse. It needs repair, as there is a significant risk of strangulation.

Easily Confused

1. Claudication and non-claudication condition

Claudication	Non-claudication condition
Pain comes on with exercise	Pain as soon as weight bears
Numbness unusual	Numbness common
Pain exacerbated by inclines or hurrying	Pain constant
	Pain around joints or feet
Pain in muscle belly (calf, thigh, buttock)	Pain may stop instantly or continue
	Pulses present
Pain disappears after a few minutes of rest	Abnormal gait
	Straight leg raising may reproduce pain
Absent pulses, diagnosis more likely	Causes: spinal canal stenosis, sciatica, osteoarthritis, muscle pathology (polymyalgia, statin-induced), neurological conditions such as motor neurone disease
Normal gait	
Straight leg raising normal	
Causes: peripheral vascular disease, popliteal aneurysms, popliteal entrapment	

2. Globus/benign dysphagia and malignant dysphagia

Globus/benign dysphagia	Malignant dysphagia
Sensation high in the neck	Symptoms lower down and vague
No regurgitation	Regurgitation
No weight loss	Weight loss
Not progressive	Progressive
Neurological symptoms	No neurological symptoms
Non-urgent referral	Needs referral under the 2-week cancer pathway

3. Inguinal hernia and femoral hernia

Inguinal hernia	Femoral hernia
More common	Less common
Often easily reduced	Usually irreducible
Above and medial to pubic tubercle	Below and lateral to the pubic tubercle

4. Appendicitis and gastroenteritis

Appendicitis	Gastroenteritis
Starts with central abdominal pain which may be constant	May have no pain or a feeling of bloating or colicky central pain; can be severe with infections such as campylobacter
Pain localises to right iliac fossa, worse on movement or coughing	Pain does not localise
Might have diarrhoea and vomiting, or constipation	Will have diarrhoea and/or vomiting as a major symptom
Other members of family or friends are well, and there is no obvious source for infection	Family and friends may have similar symptoms from an obvious source (though be careful not to jump to conclusions)
Guarding in the right iliac fossa	No guarding

Prescribing Points

1. **Acute thrombophlebitis**

   Even though associated with severe pain and a spreading inflammation, this does not require antibiotics; it is a chemically induced inflammatory response, not a bacterial one. So treatment is with NSAIDs (oral or topical), stockings and mobilisation. If the thrombophlebitis is near the saphenofemoral or saphenopopliteal junction, an ultrasound scan is required to assess the full extent. This is because there is a risk of propagation to the deep veins. Superficial thrombophlebitis is also associated with an underlying DVT (between 6% and 53%), so be vigilant for DVT.

2. **Pain relief in the acute abdomen**

   It is a myth that you cannot give analgesia to patients with an acute abdomen until they have been assessed surgically. In fact, the surgical assessment is helped enormously if pain relief is given in primary care before arrival in hospital.

3. **Antibiotics are not required for biliary colic**

   In the absence of fever or tenderness, biliary colic does not require antibiotics. Treat the pain with diclofenac or opiates such as morphine, and arrange an ultrasound.

4. **Morphine and constipation**

   Avoid morphine for chronic abdominal pain, because the constipation will produce more symptoms of pain and exacerbate the clinical picture. Refer to your local guidelines for alternatives.

5. **Post-operative wound infection**

   It is not uncommon for wounds to look a little red. There is much debate about the definition of post-operative wound infection. If there is surrounding redness (cellulitis) that is not improving or systemic symptoms, consider a wound swab and start on antibiotics. If there is fluctuance on the wound, remove the nearest clip or suture and allow the pus to drain. Take a swab. Antibiotics are not required if there is no systemic upset or spreading cellulitis. Serosanguinous (pink bloodstained fluid) that is coming from a laparotomy wound might not be a sign of infection but indicate pending dehiscence. Discuss with the surgical team.

Acknowledgements to Miss Amy Burger, Mr Jonathan Easterbrook and Mr Bhaskar Kumar for specialised advice.

GENETICS AND GENOMICS

Jude Hayward and Imran Rafi

Ten Pearls of Wisdom

1. **Genomic medicine can impact primary care in many ways and will assume increasing importance**

   Genetic issues can present to primary care in various ways. These include diseases with a possible genetic basis (see Pearl 3) and patients with a concerning family history (see Pearl 9). DNA sequencing technology has advanced significantly, enabling study of the whole genome or of coding genes described as whole-exome sequencing. Patients may even present via direct-to-consumer genetic tests (see the 'Easily confused' section). In addition, general practice IT systems can search for those at risk of or affected by inherited conditions. As we gather more information on gene variants, we will be able to clinically apply polygenic risk scores (PRS). These risk scores (also known as polygenic scores and genetic risk scores) represent the total number of genetic variants that an individual has and are used to assess their heritable risk of developing a particular disease and to assess the risk of disease alongside environmental risk. This is being researched in oncology for breast and prostate cancer, and in cardiovascular disease in primary care. Disease risk stratification will over time embed within screening programmes.

2. **Don't forget the possibility of familial hypercholesterolaemia (FH) when the total cholesterol is significantly elevated**

   Recognition of familial hypercholesterolemia in the context of raised cholesterol (www.nice.org.uk/guidance/cg71) is important because the diagnosis has a significant impact on surveillance, risk stratification and treatment. FH is an autosomal disorder with a prevalence of 1 in 250. It is characterised by alterations in genes, including those coding for the low-density lipoprotein receptor (LDLR). Affected individuals may be at risk of early heart disease, although there may be variable penetrance. A combination of raised cholesterol (TC >7.5 mmol/L, LDL >4.9 mmol/L) and signs of raised cholesterol (e.g. tendon xanthomata) or a family history of premature ischaemic heart disease (mean

 DOI: 10.1201/9781003304586-15

age of onset of coronary symptoms is 45 years in men and 55 years in women) should prompt consideration of FH. QRISK underestimates cardiovascular risk in individuals with FH; diagnosis should prompt immediate management with high-intensity lipid-lowering treatment to achieve specified targets. NICE guidelines on FH advocate cascade screening of family members including children, carried out in secondary care.

3. Know the red flags for rare genetic diseases

Recognition of red flags, rather than an in-depth knowledge of individual rare diseases, is key. In 2004, Whelan et al. devised a mnemonic of the relevant red flags: 'Family GENES'.

- *Family history*: Multiple affected siblings or individuals in multiple generations. Don't forget that a lack of a family history does not rule out genetic causes.
- *G*: Groups of congenital anomalies. Two or more anomalies are much more likely to indicate the presence of a syndrome with genetic implications.
- *E*: Extreme or exceptional presentation of common conditions. Examples are early onset of disease or unusually severe reaction to infectious or metabolic stress.
- *N*: Neurodevelopmental delay or degeneration. This would include developmental delay, developmental regression in children or early onset of neurologic deterioration in adults.
- *E*: Extreme or exceptional pathology. Examples include rare tumours or other pathology or multiple primary cancers in one or different tissues.
- *S*: Surprising laboratory values. Look for abnormal laboratory values in an otherwise healthy individual or extreme laboratory values for a typical clinical situation.

4. Be aware of the importance of family history in cancer cases

Cancer is an example of a multifactorial disease; about 5% of people diagnosed with cancer have an underlying autosomal inherited cancer predisposition syndrome such as BRCA1, BRCA2 or Lynch syndrome, with an additional 10%–15% being the above-population risk of developing cancer as a result of family history. The primary care role is to identify those at above-population risk to facilitate onward referral. At any risk level, management strategies remain the same: giving clear risk advice, discussing risk reduction options, screening, explaining symptoms of concern, advising re-attendance if the family history changes and ensuring patients are aware of whether they are eligible for genomic testing. Clear guidelines exist for some cancers (e.g. familial breast cancer, https://www.nice.org.uk/guidance /cg41). Onward referral is crucial to address risk. For example, women with Lynch syndrome may have up to a 50% lifetime risk of colorectal cancer and up to a 50% lifetime risk of endometrial cancer, which can be significantly reduced through colonoscopic screening and consideration of risk-reducing hysterectomy.

5. Cystic fibrosis has a high carrier rate – so be aware of the issues and act promptly

Cystic fibrosis (CF) is an autosomal recessive condition with a carrier frequency of 1 in 23 for northern Europeans. Couples at risk of having a child with a genetic condition such as CF may present within primary care concerned about their risk and asking about options. Urgent discussion with specialist services, preferably before pregnancy, is crucial to enable the full range of reproductive choices, including testing during pregnancy. A woman who is already pregnant and known to be a carrier for an altered CF gene may request her partner to be tested to determine the risk to the offspring. It is possible to have a prenatal diagnosis by chorionic villus sampling at 11 weeks gestation; this illustrates the need for timely and urgent referral in early pregnancy for counselling and access to reproductive choices.

6. Don't forget to refer men with actual or possible BRCA gene mutations

Patients may be offered BRCA mutation testing if they have breast cancer at an unusually young age, certain types of breast cancer at a young age, certain types of ovarian cancer, a strong family history of cancer suggesting the presence of BRCA1 or 2 mutations, or a relative with a BRCA1 or 2 mutation. Men with BRCA2 gene mutations have a higher risk of developing prostate, breast and pancreatic cancer. BRCA1 mutations in males are less of a concern, though they slightly increase the risk of breast cancer (and, possibly, prostate cancer). A pitfall is not referring a man, as autosomal dominant (AD) inheritance means there is a 50% chance of inheriting for both genders, even if a consequence is gender-specific, e.g. ovarian cancer.

7. Microarray testing can enable children to access special needs support at school

Microarray testing screens the entire genome for deletions or duplications of small numbers of DNA base pairs known as microdeletions or microduplications. These are collectively known as neurosusceptibility variants and may be associated with developmental delay, autism, epilepsy and dysmorphic features, depending on the variant. They are usually inherited in an autosomal dominant way but have a wide spectrum of clinical presentation (variable penetrance) with some individuals never being aware or displaying any symptoms or signs. They have become an important test for children previously without a genetic diagnosis. Diagnosis can, for example, open doors to access special needs support at school. Testing may be offered to parents for information purposes, but they are not generally used to inform reproductive decisions because of the extremely variable penetrance. The charity Unique publishes a disorder guide for all known micro-duplications and micro-deletions for families and healthcare professionals.

8. Understand the difference between diagnostic testing and predictive testing

Testing in an individual with symptoms of any inherited condition is known as diagnostic testing. But if a gene variant is known to run in the family, predictive testing can be offered. Huntington's disease (HD) is a good example. It is an autosomal dominant condition characterised by progressive neurodegeneration; it is 100% penetrant with significant implications for employment and insurance. The mainstay of clinical management is symptom management and supportive care. There are significant implications of having a test; predictive testing is offered but only after a series of meetings with genetic counsellors. Unaffected family members do change their minds about testing even though they may be at a 50% risk of having inherited the affected altered gene. In these situations, rare disease websites are valuable resources which carry an enormous amount of practical information for patients and healthcare professionals, and the Huntington's Disease Association (hda.org.uk) is an excellent example.

9. Know what information to provide in any referral to genetic services

Primary care has played a longstanding role in assessing risk through family histories and genetic red flags, thereby facilitating appropriate onward referral and clinical management. Patients may present with concerns regarding a genomic test result from a relative, or a family history either of a single-gene condition or conditions such as cancer or cardiovascular disease. As an increasing number of patients become eligible for genetic/genomic testing, there will be more presentations in practice with the result from a family member. Or patients may present with features which suggest a genetic disorder. It's important to provide the key points in any referral. This would include as much accurate and specific information as possible about any index case or test and a full family history. There are tools available to facilitate family history taking and recording, such as from the Genomics Education Programme (www.genomicseducation.hee.nhs.uk/taking-and-drawing-a-family-history/). Genetic specialists do use pedigree drawing software (not available for general practice IT systems) and usually draw a three-generation pedigree.

10. Support and education in genomics are readily available

Health Education England, through its Genomics Education Programme, has commissioned a programme of education that will support both general practice and secondary care. GeNotes (genomic notes for clinicians;

www.genomicseducation.hee.nhs.uk/genotes/) provides an educational resource online. A two-tier system with an introduction to topics such as oncology links to deeper knowledge areas. A GP working group has identified topics that will support GPs while they are consulting with patients. This will help GPs in managing conditions such as hereditary haemochromatosis and prostate cancer where knowledge of genomics will impact referral pathways to secondary care or allow management within primary care.

Obscure and Overlooked Diagnoses

1. **Genetic haemochromatosis**

   Causes of raised ferritin include inflammatory conditions, alcohol excess and genetic haemochromatosis (GH). GH is an example of an autosomal recessive condition, a single-gene condition which is identifiable in primary care. It is a disorder of iron metabolism that leads to progressive iron overload. Affected individuals may present with joint pains, fatigue and breathlessness. Diagnosis is crucial, as early intervention reduces later complications resulting from iron deposition in organs, for instance, in the pancreas, resulting in diabetes; within myocardial tissue, causing conduction abnormalities; and within the testes, causing subfertility. Diagnosis is made through in-depth iron studies, and referring individuals with raised transferrin saturations for genotyping. There are two common altered genes: C282Y and H63D. Disease expression is variable, so those with a genetic predisposition may not develop severe disease. First-degree relatives will need to be offered testing for identified variants.

2. **Young or unexplained cardiac death**

   Patients may present with a family history of sudden cardiac death (SCD), cardiomyopathy or arrhythmia. Testing an affected family member gives the best chance of diagnosis, with ensuing access to predictive testing for family members. Evolving testing technologies and clinical pathways are enabling the testing of tissue from deceased relatives; splenic tissue can now be utilised post-mortem for genomic testing. It is crucial that primary care facilitates access via the medical examiner pathways to appropriate testing post-mortem. Assessment usually involves testing multiple relevant genes simultaneously: 'gene panel testing'. Identifying a gene variant in affected family members gives access to targeted screening and can also identify those family members who are not at increased risk and in whom surveillance is not indicated. This can also significantly reduce anxiety and uncertainty.

3. **Neurosusceptibility variants**

   Scenarios such as 'My son has learning difficulties and epilepsy. He's about to be discharged by children's services, he's never had a diagnosis' are increasingly common. These children originally presented with symptoms many years ago and were offered only the genetic testing available at that time. The transition from paediatric to adult care provides an opportunity to revisit diagnoses and identify patients who may benefit from testing through more novel technologies. For example, these patients may be offered testing via micro-array (see Pearl 5), which can identify neurosusceptibility variants (small insertions, duplications or deletions of a few base pairs). This brings a new possibility for diagnosis which may be a powerful tool in enabling access to support for employment, living and financial support.

Easily Confused

1. **Genomic medicine and genetic medicine**
   Clinical genetics refers to the study of individual genes and inherited disorders (such as CF). Genomics is the study of the entirety of an individual's DNA, or genome, with genomic medicine being the clinical application. It is important for primary care to have an understanding of the nomenclature, as results are cascaded back from specialist care. Pathogenic gene variants are variants associated with a higher probability of being disease-causing, benign variants indicate gene variants not associated with disease causality and 'variants of uncertain clinical significance' represent gene variants that have been identified but for which evidence regarding pathogenicity is equivocal. A clinical application would be the recommendation for a risk-reducing oophorectomy in a woman carrying a BRCA1 variant. Such clinical decisions are based on pathogenic variants, not benign or variants of uncertain clinical significance.

2. **Genomic testing for gene variations within a cancer and inherited disease**
   Increasingly, genomic testing for gene variants within a cancer itself is utilised to guide cancer treatment. Mutations in the BRAF gene within melanoma mean that specific targeted therapies may be offered as a treatment choice (see NICE Guidance, 'Dabrafenib with trametinib for adjuvant treatment of resected BRAF V600 mutation-positive melanoma'). BRAF gene testing in this scenario means gene testing of the cancer itself, an example of somatic testing (testing for gene variants which are only present in a particular tissue or tissue sample). Patients may hear that their cancer is 'genetic' and assume this means it may be heritable. Germ-line variants occur in reproductive cells (egg or sperm) that become incorporated into the DNA of every cell in the body of the offspring. Germ-line variants are passed from parents to offspring and thus are heritable. Somatic variants such as in this example are non-inheritable, and family members do not need to be offered gene testing.

3. **The results of direct-to-consumer genetic tests**

Commercial companies are offering direct-to-consumer (DTC) genetic tests which may land on a GP's desk when patients present with anxiety about results and seek advice. This information may include a risk for a common multifactorial condition or that they are carriers for a gene variant within a single gene (e.g. BRCA1, cystic fibrosis). The Royal College of General Practitioners (RCGP) and the British Society for Genetic Medicine (BSGM) have a position statement regarding the results of direct-to-consumer genomic or genetic testing (www.rcgp .org.uk/representing-you/policy-areas/genomic-position-statement). In general, these patients should be managed as per usual NHS pathways, with onward referral being indicated in significant family histories or if a gene variant is found within a gene tested for within the NHS.

Prescribing Points

1. **Prescribing to reduce cancer risk**

Medications may be recommended for prescription in specific patient groups at an increased risk of specific cancers as a risk-reducing measure. For example, Lynch syndrome is a hereditary condition that primarily increases the risk of colorectal and endometrial cancers. In individuals with this syndrome, high-dose aspirin results in a 63% reduction in the relative risk of developing colorectal cancer compared with those given a placebo. Recommendations would be made by appropriate specialists (e.g. gastroenterology or clinical genetics) with a request for continuation long-term by primary care. Another example is the use of tamoxifen or anastrozole as a risk-reducing measure for women at moderate risk of developing breast cancer; again, initiation of such a prescription would be recommended via secondary care.

2. **Prescribing the combined contraceptive pill in women with a family history of breast cancer**

The UK Medical Eligibility Criteria for Contraceptive Use (UKMEC) tables remain the key reference resource in this situation. In the presence of a family history, combined hormonal contraception remains for 'unrestricted use'. All cancer risks should be balanced, discussing contraceptive risks and benefits; even if a patient is a known carrier of a gene mutation associated with cancer (BRCA1), combined hormonal contraception is still 'only' a risk category 3 (requiring expert clinical judgement). A common pitfall is to decline prescriptions without seeking expert advice; such women also have a significant lifetime risk of ovarian cancer, which may be reduced by the combined hormonal contraceptive.

3. Gene testing directing routine medication

In the next 5 to 10 years, the use of genomic data to guide prescribing (pharmacogenomics) is likely to be implemented in the NHS. There is evidence that variants in genes involved in drug metabolism or response affect the efficacy and the likelihood of an adverse drug response. One example is the use of aspirin and dipyridamole instead of clopidogrel because of gene testing in a post-CVA patient showing the patient is a CYP2C19-poor metaboliser, meaning clopidogrel would be less effective in secondary prevention. Virtually 100% of people carry a gene variant which affects drug response. The commonest medications affected are psychiatric (including SSRIs), cardiac (clopidogrel, statins), gastrointestinal (PPIs) and analgesic agents (opioids). In primary care, many patients are prescribed multiple medications (polypharmacy), and the use of pharmacogenomic testing has the potential to address inappropriate polypharmacy, non-concordance, adverse drug reactions and medication costs. Soon, we may well be prescribing medications taking genomics into account with clinical decision support systems which incorporate relevant prescribing guidance at the point of care.

GYNAECOLOGY

Elizabeth Ball and Adam Rosenthal

Ten Pearls of Wisdom

1. **Beware that patients with PCOS are at risk of metabolic disorder and endometrial cancer**

   Any two of oligomenorrhoea, hyperandrogenism or polycystic ovaries on scan can lead to a diagnosis of polycystic ovary syndrome (PCOS). Due to the long-term metabolic risk, PCOS patients require yearly checks for glucose intolerance, hypertension and dyslipidaemia, and lifestyle advice. A 10% loss in BMI often regulates ovulation. As a rule, PCOS patients should not go beyond 4 months without menstruation because of the risk of endometrial hyperplasia or cancer, which can be prevented by using a combined oral contraceptive, cyclical progestogen or the levonorgestrel intrauterine system.

2. **First-line treatment of stress and mixed urinary incontinence is weight loss and physiotherapy**

   Before considering referral, medication or surgery, these women should try to lose weight if their BMI is greater than 30. This might alleviate incontinence and increase the response to medical and surgical interventions. They should have physiotherapy sessions learning pelvic floor muscle training for at least 3 months, and then continue doing at least eight contractions three times per day.

3. **Most cases of abdominal pain in pregnancy are harmless – but don't miss abruption, preterm labour and appendicitis**

   Common causes of pain include stretching of the round ligaments, typically in the second trimester, and musculoskeletal pain from altered body posture.

   But be sure to palpate the uterus: it may help distinguish obstetric from non-obstetric pain. You may be able to palpate contractions. If these do not settle within an hour, the patient may be in premature labour; other clues are vaginal blood and mucus loss. Bear in mind that a UTI is a common cause of both abdominal pain in pregnancy and preterm labour. A tender and tense uterus on palpation with or without vaginal bleeding indicates abruption; refer without delay, especially after the gestation of viability (24–26 weeks). And remember non-obstetric causes: appendicitis affects 1:1000 pregnancies and commonly

DOI: 10.1201/9781003304586-16

presents with fever, nausea and right-lower-quadrant pain. Upward displacement of the appendix can lead to pain perceived more cranially, misleading the unwary. Beware that increased abdominal wall tension in pregnancy can mask peritonism.

4. In persistent and/or worsening intra-abdominal symptoms, think ovarian cancer

Ovarian cancer is relatively uncommon, whereas its typical symptoms are very common. No wonder that patients and their families frequently complain of long delays in diagnosis. Persistent and/or worsening of intra-abdominal symptoms should ring alarm bells – 'persistent' meaning on most days for at least 3 weeks. Irritable bowel syndrome (IBS) is rarely a correct new diagnosis in postmenopausal women. Bear in mind that a normal CA125 does not rule out ovarian cancer, so women with persistent pelvic/lower abdominal pain, abdominal distension/bloating and feeling full quickly after eating/nausea (and more rarely, change in bowel and bladder habits or lower back pain) should undergo a transvaginal ultrasound. Risk groups are postmenopausal women, those with a family history of ovarian and/or breast cancer, and those with Ashkenazi (Eastern European) Jewish heritage.

5. Have a low threshold for examining women who complain of vulval itch with no other symptoms

This symptom can result from vulval pre-malignancy. Lichen sclerosus (LS) and vulval intra-epithelial neoplasia (VIN) can both present with vulval itching/discomfort and are associated with a long-term risk of vulval squamous cell carcinoma (VSCC), so examination of patients with these symptoms is important. LS causes classic appearances of loss of normal vulval architecture (predominantly resorption of labia minora), and hyperkeratosis and pallor in a figure-of-eight distribution around the vulva and anus. It is treated with potent topical steroids, which should be initiated by a specialist.

'Usual type VIN' usually appears as discrete raised patches of white, brown or red skin. 'Differentiated VIN' tends to appear as a discrete thickened white plaque on a background of LS changes. The presence of ulceration raises the possibility of cancer.

6. Severe endometriosis requires early diagnosis

In primary care, there can be difficulties and delays in making the diagnosis of endometriosis, which can lead to loss of income, quality of life and chances of having a baby. Look out for women who only respond partially to hormones, have severe dyspareunia and pain on defecation or suffer fertility problems. Other pointers are deep endometriosis 'hotspots' that can be felt as retro-cervical induration on vaginal examination, often combined with a retroverted uterus.

A routine transvaginal ultrasound scan cannot rule out deeply infiltrating endometriosis but may show a retroverted uterus and ovarian endometrioma. Women with more severe endometriosis are the ones most likely to benefit from surgery, but this can be technically challenging and often requires a multidisciplinary team setup. Because response is best to the first surgery, it is important to get this right. Endometriosis care is now centralised in accredited endometriosis centres (http://bsge.org.uk/centre/).

7. Endometrial cancer before menopause can easily be overlooked

We recognise postmenopausal bleeding (PMB) as a red flag for endometrial cancer, but endometrial cancer or hyperplasia (which can be premalignant) can also occur in premenopausal women, especially those with risk factors (PCOS, obesity, strong family history of endometrial/bowel/ovarian cancer). Owing to cyclical changes in the endometrium, a premenopausal ultrasound is unreliable for ruling out neoplasia. Therefore, women with persistent intermenstrual bleeding over the age of 40 (or younger if risk factors are present) should be considered for endometrial biopsy. This can be done in primary care using endometrial aspiration, which must enter the uterine cavity for adequate sampling.

8. Teenage girls with 'period problems' need to be taken seriously – they may have pelvic pathology

Previously, it was thought that endometriosis and adenomyosis causing secondary dysmenorrhoea only affect women in their third or fourth decade. The increasing availability and sophistication of ultrasound scanning have shown that these conditions exist in teenagers, too. Endometriosis and adenomyosis often respond well to hormones such as COC combined oral contraceptive pill (COC) and progesterones such as the progesterone-only pill (POP), Depo-Provera, implants and intra-uterine systems (IUSs). However, many severe cases of endometriosis still go underdiagnosed and undertreated for many years, hence diminishing the chances of successful surgery and fertility treatment.

9. Chronic pelvic pain (CPP) requires a multipronged approach

This condition may have structural, functional and psychological aspects:

a. *Heavy menstrual bleeding (HMB)*: In conjunction with pelvic pain, this may suggest adenomyosis, endometriosis or both. If fibroids are the cause of HMB, they usually cause pressure symptoms, depending on their location, rather than pain.

b. *'Sensitive bowels'*: Many CPP patients with or without endometriosis complain of symptoms of IBS. Dietary adjustments such as the low FODMAP diet, mebeverine, and treatment of constipation and diarrhoea can bring relief.

c. *Depression and fatigue*: These are features of many chronic pain syndromes. CBT and mindfulness training have been shown to help, especially for depression associated with chronic pain.

d. *Subfertility*: Due to the higher incidence of structural pelvic problems in CPP patients, fertility referral should be early, especially in women over 35 years old.

e. *Deep dyspareunia*: The Ohnut sexual aid consists of four stretchy polymer blend rings worn on the base of the penis to act as a buffer. The rings can be stacked to control the depth of penetration during intercourse.

f. *Myofascial pelvic pain*: Often co-exists with other pathology, but is often underdiagnosed. Symptoms can include piercing clitoral and rectal pain, but pain may also be described as 'achy' and be either constant or intermittent. Assessment including checking for trigger points, and treatment is usually carried out by a specially qualified physiotherapist.

10. For a 'state-of-the-art HRT regime' consider combining the Mirena IUS with transdermal oestrogen

The benefits of transdermal oestrogen include more stable serum oestradiol levels, less effect on liver metabolism, less hypercoagulation and fewer 'metabolic syndrome'-type side effects, with better bioavailability of the metabolite testosterone. Straightforward endometrial protection is delivered by levonorgestrel from the IUS. Many women will already have an in-date IUS when they reach menopause, which will continue to protect against pregnancy in the perimenopausal years. If the IUS is used as part of HRT, it should be changed every 4 years, not every 5 years.

Obscure or Overlooked Diagnoses

1. **Painful bladder syndrome (PBS)**

   PBS (formerly interstitial cystitis) overlaps with symptoms of endometriosis, such as cyclical exacerbation of pelvic pain and dyspareunia. In fact, these 'ugly twins' often co-exist. Always consider PBS in a pelvic pain patient with nocturia and a 'negative laparoscopy'. The triad of bladder filling pain, frequent nocturia and bladder base tenderness (on vaginal examination) is highly suggestive. Clearly, UTI should be ruled out. There is debate whether this syndrome should be diagnosed just from the clinical history, or whether cystoscopy under general anaesthesia and distending the bladder with water – thereby provoking petechial bleeds secondary to a damaged bladder lining – is needed. Several treatments have been tried (physiotherapy, amitriptyline, gabapentin and instillation with botulinum toxin).

2. **Endometriosis outside the pelvic cavity**

   a. *Abdominal wall endometriosis*: This usually develops in surgical scars resulting from a caesarean section or from a laparoscopic port site. It often co-exists with pelvic endometriosis but may occur in isolation.

    b. *Sciatic nerve endometriosis*: Endometriosis can infiltrate the area around pelvic nerves/the sacral plexus causing pudendal and gluteal pain, sciatic neuralgia and other neurological symptoms.

    c. *Thoracic endometriosis*: Recurrent pneumothorax and haemoptysis during menstrual periods can point towards endometriosis affecting the tracheobronchial tree, lung parenchyma and lung pleura.

3. **Pudendal nerve entrapment**

   Anoperineal pain, especially the inability to sit comfortably, may point towards entrapment of the pudendal nerve, which supplies the sensation to the pelvic area and motor function to the pelvic floor muscles and urethral sphincter. CT-guided local anaesthetic applied close to the ischial spine aids diagnosis. Surgery to decompress the pudendal nerve can help.

4. ***Actinomyces* and intra-uterine contraception**

   Actinomyces, a gram-positive anaerobic bacillus, is part of the normal flora. Its presence in a smear test or in the vagina is not predictive of any possible complications such as endometritis, PID or pelvic abscesses. If it is found in smears of asymptomatic women, it probably represents colonisation, so treatment or IUD removal is not required. In the presence of clinical evidence of pelvic infection, antibiotics should be administered according to local antimicrobial recommendations and the IUD removed. The IUS has a lower incidence of *Actinomyces* on cervical smears than copper IUDs, where it can be present in 7% of smears.

Easily Confused

1. **Cervical ectopy/ectropion (previous erosion) and cervical cancer**

Cervical ectopy/ectropion (previously erosion)	Cervical cancer
■ Associated with postcoital bleeding and heavy, clear discharge	■ Even early stages can present with abnormal bleeding (postcoital, intermenstrual, postmenopausal) and foul discharge
■ Diagnosis made on speculum examination ± colposcopy if any concern about cancer or need for treatment of symptoms	■ Diagnosis made on biopsy following referral to rapid access clinic for abnormal appearance of cervix; occasionally diagnosed as a result of abnormal smear
■ Not usually associated with other gynaecological symptoms	■ Pelvic or leg pain, lymphoedema, haematuria, uraemia and fistulae are signs of advanced disease
■ Common, especially in younger women on the combined pill	■ Rare in those who have attended for regular smears, especially if most recent is HPV negative; have higher index of suspicion in immigrants from countries with no screening, e.g. Africa, Asia, Eastern Europe

2. Endometrial polyp and endometrial hyperplasia

Endometrial polyp	Endometrial hyperplasia
■ Incidental finding or presenting with heavy and prolonged menstrual bleeding	■ Oligomenorrhoea followed by heavy bleeding, prolonged or intermenstrual bleeding ■ Risk factors are PCOS and high BMI
■ Low malignant potential if asymptomatic ■ Diagnosis with Aquascan or hysteroscopy; scan may only show thickened endometrium ■ Treatment with biopsy or hysteroscopic removal	■ High malignant potential if atypical hyperplasia is present ■ Diagnosis with ultrasound scan and endometrial biopsy ■ Treatment depending on severity, age, parity with Mirena IUS or hysterectomy

3. Adenomyosis and fibroids

Adenomyosis	Fibroids
■ Heavy painful periods, dragging pelvic sensation, chronic pelvic pain ■ Examination reveals 'boggy', painful uterus ■ Progesterone, especially IUS, often cures the pain; hysterectomy only in refractory cases and when family is complete	■ Heavy periods, and pressure on bowel and bladder usually more prominent than pain ■ Firm enlarged uterus, subserosal fibroids can sometimes be palpated distinctly ■ Dependent on symptoms and fibroid position, Mirena can help with HMB; surgical options include hysteroscopic, laparoscopic and open surgery with removal of fibroids or uterus

Prescribing Points

1. **Tranexamic acid**

   Taken regularly during menses (or ideally the night before), this can reduce flow by 50%. It was originally used for bleeding in von Willebrand's disease, but it helps in menorrhagia, whether caused by von Willebrand's or not. There is an additive effect when used together with mefenamic acid. Unfortunately, patients often underdose or get confused because of the similar names. The correct doses are mefenamic acid, 500 mg three times daily (narrow therapeutic window, overdosage can cause convulsions); and tranexamic acid, 1 g three times daily for up to 4 days, which can be increased to 4 g daily.

2. **Low-dose aspirin in pregnancy**

   In women at high risk of pre-eclampsia (e.g. previous pre-eclampsia, diabetes, chronic renal disease, chronic hypertension), 75 mg aspirin per day given from week 12 can help reduce the risks of hypertensive disorders in pregnancy and therefore improve the chances of a healthy baby. A combination of moderate risk factors also justifies this approach, but its use in the prevention of miscarriage is not supported by the evidence.

3. **Oral hyoscine butylbromide**

   This antispasmodic is often prescribed for smooth muscle cramps in IBS and dysmenorrhoea. Owing to its chemical structure (ammonium bonds), oral bioavailability is very poor and patients who may recall effective pain relief after parenteral administration may not respond to oral treatment.

4. **Vaginal micronised progesterone**

   For women in early pregnancy with a scan-confirmed intrauterine pregnancy with a fetal heartbeat who have previously had at least one miscarriage and are experiencing vaginal bleeding, offer vaginal micronised progesterone 400 mg twice a day up to 16 weeks of pregnancy. The initial prescription should be provided by the early pregnancy unit and the ongoing prescribing taken up by the woman's GP.

HAEMATOLOGY

Andy Hughes

Ten Pearls of Wisdom

1. With anaemia, the MCV is the most useful initial guide to causation

Microcytosis suggests iron deficiency (but see Pearl 2). Mild iron deficiency can be confused with thalassaemia trait, but the latter has a very low mean corpuscular volume (MCV) and may have a suggestive ethnic background (see the section 'Easily confused'). The anaemia of chronic disease can be microcytic in approximately 25% of patients. Macrocytosis suggests B_{12} or folate deficiency, and in the older patient may indicate myelodysplasia. Macrocytosis, with or without anaemia, can also be seen with liver disease, haemolysis and hypothyroidism. Macrocytosis with a normal Hb can reflect excess alcohol consumption. A normal MCV with low white cells or platelets in the context of anaemia may suggest an underlying bone marrow disorder.

2. Iron deficiency may still be the cause of anaemia, even with a normal MCV and ferritin – especially in the elderly

Forty percent of individuals with iron deficiency anaemia may have a normal MCV. The sensitivity of a low ferritin of <15 µg/L for iron deficiency is only 59%, but 98% if <40 µg/L. The transferrin (iron) saturation (Tsat) is a useful test in these circumstances. This is widely available but usually only carried out for high ferritin levels. If the Tsat is <15%, then it is likely that the individual is iron deficient. If in doubt, and a Tsat is not available, a short 4–6 week trial of oral iron is worthwhile.

3. Not all low B_{12} results mean true deficiency

The B_{12} assay is not very sensitive or specific. Borderline low levels (up to 25% below the local reference range) may not equate with true deficiency. Falsely normal levels can also occur. Clinical features such as glossitis, paraesthesia, unsteadiness or peripheral neuropathy, especially loss of proprioception or vibration sense, make true deficiency more likely. A macrocytic anaemia, especially with an MCV of >110 fl, and hypersegmented polymorphs on a blood film are also suggestive of true deficiency. If in doubt, repeat testing in 1 or 2

DOI: 10.1201/9781003304586-17

months can be useful, with a persistently low or progressively decreasing B_{12} indicative of true deficiency. With a suggestive clinical picture, a trial of B_{12} can be given, even if the B_{12} level is normal.

4. Leucocytosis is not always due to infection

Benign, non-infectious causes of leucocytosis are usually mild, long-standing, non-progressive and not associated with other full blood count (FBC) abnormalities. In primary care, persistent leucocytosis with neutrophilia and occasionally monocytosis is most commonly associated with smoking, which may persist for years after smoking cessation. Obesity can also be associated with leucocytosis, especially in females. High-dose steroids or a previous splenectomy are other possible causes. Persistent unexplained lymphocytosis, especially in those over 65, should raise suspicion of chronic lymphatic leukaemia.

5. Long-standing neutropenia is likely to be benign

Long-standing, isolated, non-progressive neutropenia is usually benign and does not generally require referral. In Afro-Caribbean patients, it is probably benign ethnic neutropenia. Neutropenia may be autoimmune and can be associated with other autoimmune disorders, such as lupus. B_{12} or folate deficiency can also cause neutropenia. Regular FBCs are usually not necessary and should be done only if there is a good clinical reason. Infection risk only really begins to increase with neutrophils of $<0.5 \times 10^9$/L. Recent, unexplained neutropenia, especially if progressive, less than 0.5×10^9/L or associated with other cytopenias, should lead to an urgent haematology referral.

Similarly, mild to moderate lymphopenia ($0.5–1.5 \times 10^9$/L) in asymptomatic individuals over 65 years old is usually benign and may be age-related. It rarely needs further investigation. Infections, including HIV and COVID-19, immunosuppression (e.g. with steroids), and surgery may all be causes of lymphopenia.

6. In most cases of mild bruising or bleeding, the history is more informative than laboratory tests

Most of these cases are benign. Single-site bleeding, such as nosebleeds or menorrhagia, is usually due to a local problem. Persistent or recurrent bleeding without a local cause may be due to a coagulation abnormality such as von Willebrand's disease with menorrhagia. Extensive, non-traumatic bruising, multiple-site bleeding, excessive bleeding from cuts, previous trauma, surgery, dental extractions, childbirth and/or a family history of excessive bruising or bleeding suggest a coagulation abnormality. Bruising on the forearms and hands in the elderly is probably age-related and can be made worse by steroids, anticoagulants, aspirin, clopidogrel and NSAIDs. Mild bruising in young women, especially confined to the limbs, is usually benign. The best initial screening tests are a platelet count, prothrombin time (PT) and activated partial thromboplastin time (aPTT), though these may be normal with mild abnormalities.

7. Most thrombocytopenia in general practice do not require a referral

While acute, severe thrombocytopenia (platelets $<20 \times 10^9$/L) should be urgently referred, most thrombocytopenia in primary care is mild to moderate, $>50 \times 10^9$/L, and does not require referral. Consider autoimmune thrombocytopenia (AITP) or secondary to other autoimmune diseases such as lupus. Consider HIV in at-risk groups, antiphospholipid syndrome and chronic liver disease (CLD), especially associated with obesity, alcohol or hepatitis. Alcohol alone can cause thrombocytopenia with a direct toxic effect on the bone marrow. Thrombocytopenia is generally mild ($100-150 \times 10^9$/L) and is rarely $<50 \times 10^9$/L. Most patients can be monitored in the community, with referral if the platelets are $<50 \times 10^9$/L or there are problems with bleeding or an associated unexplained anaemia or neutropenia.

8. Most common cause of raised ferritin is reactive

Reactive causes of a raised ferritin include infection, inflammation, metastatic malignancy or liver disease, especially if the latter is associated with excess alcohol. With a raised ferritin, a fasting Tsat should be done. A normal Tsat suggests a reactive cause, while a raised Tsat usually indicates iron overload as seen with, for example, hereditary haemochromatosis (HH). A Tsat of $>50\%$ in women and $>60\%$ in men detect $>90\%$ of individuals with HH and should lead to genetic blood testing for HH.

9. Context is everything

When assessing an individual abnormal result, previous results can determine its significance and the need for further investigation or formal referral. A rapid drop in Hb usually causes symptoms and suggests bleeding, while, with a slow decrease, patients may be asymptomatic, even at very low Hb levels. Mild, isolated, persistent and non-progressive abnormalities are rarely as significant as recent, progressive ones. Multiple FBC abnormalities are usually significant. Context includes relevant clinical features, ethnic background and personal details such as weight, smoking and alcohol habits.

10. Know how to interpret common blood film abnormalities

When there are FBC abnormalities without an obvious explanation, requesting a blood film – if not already provided by the lab – can provide simple, inexpensive, additional information about haematological disorders. Useful red blood cell abnormalities include pencil cells in iron deficiency, polychromasia indicating a raised reticulocyte response in bleeding or haemolysis, target cells in liver disease and haemoglobinopathies, and crenated cells in renal failure (although these can be artefactual). With white blood cells (WBCs), a left shift and toxic granulation are associated with infection, hypersegmented neutrophils suggest B_{12} or folate deficiency, hypogranular or bilobed neutrophils (Pelger cells) can be seen with myelodysplasia, and, with a lymphocytosis, smear cells are associated with chronic lymphatic leukaemia. Platelet aggregates or clumps are harmless *in vitro* artefacts that can be causes of a falsely low platelet count.

Obscure or Overlooked Diagnoses

1. **Haematological malignancies**
   Only six or seven patients per average size practice per year are diagnosed with haematological malignancies. The most common, especially in those over 60, are lymphomas, chronic lymphatic leukaemia, myeloma and monoclonal gammopathy of undetermined significance (MGUS), the latter being a clonal disorder with malignant potential. Suggestive features include unexplained weight loss, fever, drenching night sweats, non-tender lymphadenopathy, splenomegaly, and new bone or back pain. Suggestive blood tests include recent, unexplained cytopenias, especially pancytopenia, blood films containing blasts or that are leucoerythroblastic (presence of nucleated RBCs and immature WBCs), lymphocytosis, new hypercalcaemia or renal failure.

2. **Coeliac disease and angiodysplasia**
   While iron deficiency is commonly due to menorrhagia or gastrointestinal bleeding, it can also be due to malabsorption, as in coeliac disease, where the combination of iron and folate deficiency is suggestive. Up to 10% of gastrointestinal bleeding is from the small bowel, which is not amenable to endoscopy. The most common source is from dilated, tortuous, thin-walled blood vessels: angiodysplasia. Patients with normal endoscopies should be considered for small bowel studies.

3. **Haemolytic anaemias**
   Haemolytic anaemias are rarely seen in primary care. Consider in individuals with anaemia and jaundice but otherwise normal liver function tests (LFTs), or with a family history, as with hereditary spherocytosis. The best additional blood tests are reticulocytes and lactate dehydrogenase (LDH), the latter released from haemolysed red cells. Both are raised in haemolysis.

4. **Red cell distribution width (RDW)**
   An RDW test is a quantitative measure of the degree of variation in red cell size (anisocytosis). It is typically raised in haematinic deficiencies and may be raised in early deficiency when the MCV is normal. It may help in distinguishing iron

deficiency (raised) from thalassaemia trait (normal), or B_{12} and folate deficiencies (raised) from other causes of macrocytic anaemias (normal).

5. **Antiphospholipid syndrome**

   Antiphospholipid syndrome is associated with early or late pregnancy loss and an increased risk of arterial or venous thrombosis. It can also present with thrombocytopenia or a prolonged aPTT. Diagnostic tests include lupus anticoagulant and anticardiolipin and beta-2 glycoprotein 1 antibodies. With antibodies, usually only moderate to high levels are significant (>40 units). A firm diagnosis can only be made if positive tests remain positive on retesting after 12 weeks.

6. **Benign abnormalities in pregnancy**

   Some haematological abnormalities seen in pregnancy are benign: (a) leucocytosis up to $16 \times 10^9/L$ can occur without evidence of infection; (b) a mild fall in platelets in the second and third trimester, rarely $<70 \times 10^9/L$, gestational thrombocytopenia; (c) an increased MCV; and (d) low B_{12} (levels >25% below the laboratory low limit of normal, macrocytic anaemia, a positive intrinsic factor antibody test or clinical symptoms such as glottis, paraesthesia or peripheral neuropathy could all warrant treatment, but there is no convincing evidence that an isolated low B_{12} level in pregnancy reflects genuine deficiency).

7. **Some overlooked causes of low B_{12}**

   (a) Decreased gastric acid production associated with age-related atrophic gastritis (intrinsic factor antibody negative pernicious anaemia) and chronic proton pump inhibitor treatment; (b) terminal ileal malabsorption due to metformin; (c) post bariatric surgery; and (d) vegans and strict vegetarians, especially during pregnancy and breastfeeding.

8. **Thrombocytosis and cancer**

   An isolated thrombocytosis, e.g. $>450 \times 10^9/L$, can be associated with an underlying cancer, especially lung, endometrial and gastrointestinal. Patients should be assessed at least clinically in primary care, but one-third of patients with thrombocytosis and cancer may be asymptomatic. Referral for further investigation should be considered, especially if there is no obvious underlying cause (see later) and the thrombocytosis persists after 6 months. Thrombocytosis can also be seen in iron deficiency, following splenectomy and with acute or chronic infection or inflammation. An associated anaemia, leucocytosis or splenomegaly might suggest a myeloproliferative disorder.

9. **With idiopathic DVT and PE consider an underlying cancer but don't overinvestigate**

   About 5%–10% of individuals who sustain a DVT or PE with no obvious underlying cause are diagnosed with a malignancy within 12 months. Further investigations should be guided by a clinical assessment for suspicious symptoms or signs. Routine invasive investigations carry no significant advantages.

Easily Confused

1. Iron deficiency and thalassaemia trait

Iron deficiency	Thalassaemia trait
■ Decreased Hb	■ Hb mildly decreased or normal
■ Modest decrease in MCV	■ Marked decrease in MCV
■ Decreased ferritin	■ Normal ferritin
■ Other features:	■ Other features:
■ Decreased MCH and MCHC	■ Decreased MCH; normal or slightly decreased MCHC
■ Decreased RBCs	■ Normal or increased RBCs
■ Increased RDW	■ Normal RDW
	■ Haemoglobinopathy screening:
	■ HbA_2 increased with beta-thalassaemia trait
	■ HbA_2 normal with alpha-thalassaemia trait
	■ Suggestive ethnic origin

2. MGUS (monoclonal gammopathy of undetermined significance) and myeloma

MGUS	Myeloma
■ Low-concentration paraprotein	■ High-concentration paraprotein; usually >30 g/L; myeloma usually associated with IgG and IgA paraproteins
■ IgG <20 g/L	
■ IgA <15 g/L	
■ IgM <5 g/L	■ Other immunoglobulins may be decreased
■ Other immunoglobulins normal	
■ Patient asymptomatic	■ Suspicious symptoms and signs may be present:
	■ New onset bone pain
	■ Weight loss; fatigue
■ Hb, creatinine and calcium usually normal	■ Hb can be decreased
	■ Creatinine and calcium can be increased
■ Urine negative for Bence Jones protein (BJP)	■ Urine may be positive for Bence Jones protein (BJP)
■ No lytic lesions on X-rays	■ X-rays may show lytic lesions
Action:	Action:
■ Follow-up 6 monthly in the community	■ 2 ww referral to haematology
■ Refer with increasing paraprotein level plus:	
■ Symptomatic	
■ Unexplained anaemia	
■ Deteriorating renal function	
■ Hypercalcaemia	

3. Primary polycythaemia and secondary polycythaemia

Primary polycythaemia	Secondary polycythaemia

■ Suggestive symptoms:
  ■ Itching after baths/showers
  ■ Gout
  ■ Burning pain in hands/feet (erythromelalgia)
  ■ Arterial/venous thrombosis
  ■ Splenomegaly (c. 50%)
	■ Caused by:
	  ■ Smoking
	  ■ History of COPD
	  ■ Obesity with obstructive sleep apnoea
	  ■ Treatment with diuretics

■ FBC may show leucocytosis and/or thrombocytosis
■ Abdominal ultrasound scan:
  ■ May show splenomegaly
	■ WBCs and platelet counts usually normal
	■ Abdominal ultrasound scan:
	  ■ No splenomegaly
	  ■ Renal abnormalities
	    ■ Cysts
	    ■ Cancer (rare)

■ Blood test for JAK2[a] mutation positive in >95%	■ JAK2 negative

[a] JAK2 is a specialised blood test that haematology departments may agree to perform without a specific outpatient referral.

4. Benign lymphadenopathy and malignant lymphadenopathy

Benign lymphadenopathy	Malignant lymphadenopathy

■ Localised
  ■ Underlying local cause (e.g. infection)
  ■ Usually resolves within 4–6 weeks
	■ Generalised
	  ■ If local, there is no obvious underlying cause and doesn't resolve, or shows progressive enlargement

■ Tender
  ■ Mobile
  ■ <1 cm
	■ Non-tender
	  ■ Fixed
	  ■ Hard or rubbery

■ Local symptoms or asymptomatic	■ Systemic symptoms with fever, weight loss, drenching night sweats

Prescribing Points

1. Oral iron

Only use with proven iron deficiency (low ferritin or transferrin saturation). Using a full therapeutic dose can be associated with an incidence of gastrointestinal (GI) side effects of 30%–40%. The use of lower doses, e.g. once daily or on alternate days, has similar effectiveness but a lower rate of GI side effects. Take in the morning on an empty stomach and avoid tea (decreases absorption). Consider adding vitamin C to increase absorption. Check the Hb response after a month, and Hb and ferritin after 3 months. Failure to respond can be associated with poor patient compliance; malabsorption; continuation of the underlying cause (usually bleeding); or coexisting, active conditions such as infection, inflammation, cancer or renal failure. With genuine intolerance, malabsorption, inflammatory bowel disease, or in the third trimester of pregnancy, consider referral for intravenous iron.

2. **Monitoring non-vitamin K oral anticoagulants (DOACs)**

   Patients should be seen 1 and 3 months after initiation to check on initial tolerance, side effects, bleeding and, importantly, compliance. Then they should be seen 6–12 monthly for follow-up. If renal function is normal, then this should be checked yearly, 6 monthly if the calculated creatinine clearance (not eGFR; use online or embedded calculator, e.g. MD + Calc) is 30–60 mL/min and 3 monthly if <30 mL/min. Dose adjustments should be made according to BNF guidelines. There is no place for routine coagulation testing in primary care, unlike the use of the INR with warfarin.

3. **When should an antiplatelet agent (APA) be given or continued when oral anticoagulation (OAC) is also indicated?**

   - For the first 12 months following a myocardial infarction (MI) treated medically or following percutaneous coronary intervention (PCI) with coronary artery stent insertion.
   - After coronary artery bypass grafts, although after 1 year an APA may not be necessary after an internal mammary artery graft.
   - If an OAC is required, an existing APA can be stopped if it is being used for peripheral arterial disease, a previous stroke not related to atrial fibrillation, an MI sustained more than 12 months previously with stable ischaemic heart disease, or an MI treated with PCI more than 12 months previously.

   If in doubt about stopping an APA, it may be wise to check with the patient's cardiologist first.

4. **Anticoagulation for venous thromboembolism (VTE)**

   DOACs are now the anticoagulant of choice: they have the same efficacy as low molecular weight heparin and warfarin but are safer with less risk of bleeding. In general, VTEs provoked by COCP, pregnancy, surgery, hospital admission, immobility or long-haul plane flight need only 3 months of anticoagulation. Unprovoked VTEs, especially in men, have a higher risk of recurrence and long-term anticoagulation should be considered.

5. **Metformin and low B$_{12}$ levels**

   Metformin treatment for type-2 diabetes can decrease B$_{12}$ absorption in the terminal ileum and can be associated with low B$_{12}$ levels. The significance of this and its management remains the subject of ongoing research. Low B$_{12}$ levels have been associated with high-dose (>1500 mg/day) metformin, treatment for >5 years, patient age >65 years, and the concomitant use of protein pump inhibitors (PPIs) or H$_2$ receptor antagonists such as ranitidine. It may be useful to check a B_{12} level as a baseline at the initiation of metformin treatment, but currently, the routine checking of B_{12} levels during treatment is not recommended except perhaps if other risk factors for B_{12} deficiency exist (see earlier). B_{12} levels should be checked in the presence of unexplained anaemia, especially if macrocytic, and in the presence of suspicious clinical symptoms such as glossitis, ataxia, paraesthesia or other signs of peripheral neuropathy. With demonstrably low levels, treatment with parenteral B_{12} can be given and continued as per standard guidelines. Lowering the metformin dose could be considered. Calcium supplements have also been shown to reverse B_{12} malabsorption, as absorption appears calcium-dependent. However, routine use of calcium supplements in these circumstances is not yet recommended.

NEUROLOGY

Richard Davenport

Ten Pearls of Wisdom

1. **Sensory symptoms are very common and usually harmless**
   Numbness, tingling, and pins and needles – with or without pain – are
   exceedingly common, usually entirely benign and a specific cause is often
   difficult to identify. The most common 'trapped nerves' are the median nerve
   (lateral hand, although notoriously ignores anatomical boundaries), ulnar (ring
   and little fingers) and lateral cutaneous nerve of the thigh (obvious). Most
   patients presenting with sensory disturbance, especially if intermittent, need
   reassurance, not referral. Numb/tingling feet in older people may warrant a blood
   screen (beware the incidental low normal B_{12}) for treatable causes of neuropathy
   but rarely leads to disability. Remember also to ask about alcohol intake.

2. **Most headaches do not indicate sinister disease**
   Although headaches cause much misery for patients, very few are harbouring
   anything sinister. Don't worry too much about brain tumours – they are rare,
   generally incurable and rarely cause isolated headaches. Instead, concentrate
   on accurately diagnosing and treating migraine (paroxysmal headaches with
   associated systemic upset), chronic daily headache (most of which is chronic
   migraine, needs diagnosis and reassurance), the occasional subarachnoid
   haemorrhage (refer immediately anyone with a headache, maximal at onset
   or within minutes, lasting longer than 1 hour) and temporal arteritis (always
   over 60 years old, usually much older, look and feel awful). Remember
   mechanical neck disorders and depression commonly cause headaches, but stable
   hypertension does not, however 'logical' such a theory appears. Sinusitis causes
   acute facial pain with other infective symptoms, not chronic headaches. And
   suggesting an eye test may be a good way to end a consultation, but rarely will
   explain your patient's symptoms.

3. **'Post-concussion syndrome' does not indicate brain damage**
   People may develop a constellation of symptoms after minor head injury
   including headache, fatigue, dizziness, poor concentration/memory,
   emotionalism and numerous others. These are not specific to head injury and

DOI: 10.1201/9781003304586-18

the label of 'post-concussion syndrome' is misleading. They are often persistent and may get worse, especially if the diagnosis is not explained. Identify and treat BPPV, which is often preceded by head injury (see Pearl 5) and depression, but otherwise manage as for other functional symptoms (www.headinjurysymptoms .org/). The symptoms are very similar to other 'post-' syndromes including most recently post-COVID.

4. Beware of medication overuse headache (MOH)

All analgesics (including triptans) used to combat headaches can lead to MOH. Curiously, prolonged use of these drugs for non-head chronic pain does not cause MOH. Any headache syndrome persisting for longer than 4 weeks and not responding to simple analgesia is unlikely to be helped by increasing the level of analgesia. It is better to consider the diagnosis and treat appropriately (migraine, depression, cluster and so on). Most episodic headache syndromes are migraines, which remain underdiagnosed; think of migraines as headaches plus systemic upset, whereas tension-type headache and chronic daily headache syndromes are purely headaches.

5. Vertigo usually originates in the vestibular apparatus, not the brain

Vertigo is the illusion of movement in any plane (not just spinning) and should be distinguished from 'dizziness', 'lightheadedness', 'giddiness' and so on. Acute vertigo is most commonly due to acute vestibular failure (vestibular neuronitis) – usually profoundly unpleasant and debilitating, but settles after a few days. Transient vertigo occurring in bed or on getting up is usually benign paroxysmal positional vertigo. Brain causes of vertigo are rare, with migraine being the most common. 'Cervical vertigo' is a common diagnosis in ENT clinics but does not exist. Nor does 'vertebrobasilar insufficiency'; older people may feel dizzy when looking up, but this is common and usually due to vestibular pathology, if any.

6. Know where to send patients with diplopia

Monocular diplopia (double vision arising from one eye) is almost always due to an ocular problem, whereas binocular diplopia is usually neurological. Ask patients to cover one eye, then the other. If the diplopia resolves with either eye occluded, it is binocular (and therefore needs a neurologist). If it disappears with just one of the eyes occluded (i.e. seeing double through one eye), it is monocular, which requires an ophthalmologist. And if the patient has bilateral monocular diplopia (or triplopia), it is either bilateral eye disease (possible) or functional (more likely).

7. Know how to tell tremors apart

Both arms shaking when picking up cups or cutlery is usually essential tremor (ET). Do not be misled by a family history of Parkinson's disease (PD); this may be inaccurate because a family history is far more likely in ET than PD. Head tremor is never PD, but usually either ET or dystonic tremor. One-sided tremor (usually an arm), especially at rest, and improving briefly on picking up a cup, suggests PD. Other clues may include early non-motor symptoms such as hyposmia, depression, constipation and REM sleep behavioural disorder. Always consider PD in a patient with a treatment-resistant frozen shoulder.

8. A neurological examination is rarely of benefit in primary care

The value of a neurological examination by a non-specialist is overrated. Most common neurological symptoms (headache, focal symptoms, funny turns/ blackouts) are not associated with (real) signs and most doctors never learn to examine the nervous system adequately. It is far better to concentrate on the history, which will allow you to decide whether referral is required and if so, to whom. If you must examine, make it count (e.g. if you suspect a transient ischaemic attack [TIA], take the pulse and blood pressure, but do not bother with the nervous system).

9. Imaging is unlikely to be of value in headache, neck or back pain

Pressure from patients and others in a society that increasingly attaches more importance to modern technology than careful clinical assessment is unfortunate, expensive and frequently misleading. The emergence of VOMIT (victims of modern imaging technology) is a real problem, not just an amusing acronym; we increasingly identify abnormalities we have little idea what to do with. The reassurance value of such imaging is overrated, especially if an 'incidentaloma' is identified. Instead, we should explain to patients why imaging is not indicated for these common symptoms, although it may be a battle already lost.

10. Neck/arm and back/leg pain should generally be managed conservatively

Some of these will be prolapsed intervertebral discs causing radiculopathy, although most are not. Very few need surgery (and thus imaging). Initial management should always be analgesia, physiotherapy and, above all, time. Avoid imaging and/or referring such patients; it does not help. And do not suggest nerve conduction studies will help; they rarely, if ever, do.

Obscure or Overlooked Diagnoses

1. Rare headache syndromes

a. *Trigeminal autonomic cephalalgias*: The most 'common' is cluster, but others include hemicrania continua, paroxysmal hemicrania and short-lasting unilateral headache with conjunctival injection and tearing (SUNCT). They are all characterised by unilateral head pain, usually severe, lasting seconds to hours, associated with autonomic features (eye-watering, red conjunctiva, ptosis, nasal stuffiness). Their management is different from other headache syndromes, so early identification is key (see www.ouchuk.org).

b. *Nummular headache*: A well-demarcated area, usually in the parietal region, of mild to moderate pain with or without accompanying numbness. This is benign but often resistant to medication.

c. *Hypnic headache*: Typically older patients who are recurrently awoken by headaches of mild-to-moderate severity, lasting up to 4 hours, with no other symptoms. Migraine is a more common cause of headaches arising from sleep.

d. *Post-COVID vaccine headache*: Soon after the introduction of the AstraZeneca COVID vaccine, very rare but often disastrous venous thromboembolic syndrome emerged, including cerebral venous sinus thrombosis, which often presented with headache. Most people with post-vaccine headaches are not harbouring such sinister syndromes, and after the initial cluster of cases, it has all but disappeared with refinement in vaccine guidelines.

2. **Benign hemisensory syndrome**

Very common, but not well recognised, usually affecting the left side, with tingly numbness affecting the arm/leg and sometimes ipsilateral face; may be intermittent or persistent.

3. **Orthostatic tremor**

Usually seen in older people, with unsteadiness on standing still, immediately relieved by sitting, lying or walking. Examination is usually normal, although a tremor over the quadriceps on standing may be visible. Listening over this muscle with a stethoscope may reveal the 'helicopter hum' of an audible tremor. Clonazepam may help, although treatment is often unsuccessful.

4. **Transient global amnesia (TGA)**

Patients abruptly develop profound anterograde amnesia and variable retrograde amnesia. They otherwise appear normal, but repetitively and irritatingly question, as their immediate recall is not functioning. The symptoms resolve completely after a few hours, although they remain amnesic for the attack period. It is usually isolated, occasionally recurs and requires only reassurance – TGA is not a TIA (which rarely causes isolated amnesia), but shorter-lasting attacks may be TEA (transient epileptic amnesia). Differentiating TGA versus TIA versus TEA requires a careful history (including a witness) and pattern recognition. TGA is usually a 'one-off', whereas TEA is recurrent, with shorter episodes of amnesia (usually less than 60 minutes), often on wakening.

5. **Notalgia paraesthetica**

Characterised by an irritating, itchy area of numbness over the back in a well-circumscribed area, it may wax and wane in severity but is isolated and benign.

6. **Exploding head syndrome**

Despite the name, entirely benign. Patients describe a sudden bang or explosion within the head, without pain, sometimes with a flash of light, usually as they are waking up. Although it terrifies them (and doctors who do not recognise it), it needs reassurance only. It can recur.

7. **Sleep phenomena**

   a. *Restless legs syndrome (RLS)*: Often associated with unpleasant sensory disturbance, but the hallmark is the urge to move the legs, which affords relief. Sometimes associated with low serum ferritin (always check).

   b. *Periodic limb movements of sleep*: Unlike RLS, it occurs when the patient is asleep, so it bothers the partner, not the patient, with repetitive fidgety movements.

   c. *Parasomnias*: Occur during sleep, so trouble bed partners. The non-REM parasomnias (night terrors, sleepwalking) occur in the first half of the night, and REM disorders in the second. REM sleep behavioural disorder (acting out one's dreams) is now recognised as a potential harbinger of neurodegenerative diseases, mainly Parkinson's.

   d. *Epilepsy*: Seizures may occur exclusively at night and be difficult to distinguish from parasomnias.

   e. *Sleep paralysis*: A common isolated symptom, associated with normal health, but consider narcolepsy (ask about abrupt sleep attacks and cataplexy). Patients awaken unable to move or speak, but able to breathe; typically resolves within seconds and is often terrifying.

Easily Confused

1. Reflex syncope (fainting) and epileptic convulsion

Reflex syncope (fainting)	Epileptic convulsion
▪ Typical scenario and triggers: e.g. bathroom, restaurant/eating, healthcare setting, pain, planes	▪ Any scenario and usually no triggers
	▪ Often no warning or focal onset
▪ Warning: e.g. feel faint/sick, vision dims, tinnitus/deafness	▪ Tonic cry at onset, stiffening of limbs with arms flexed, legs extended, blue/purple colour, then clonic phase, usually 1–2 mins, blood/foam from mouth
▪ Witness: brief loss of consciousness, pale, still, sweaty, may have brief stiffening, myoclonic jerks	▪ Enter deep sleep with heavy snoring, gradual recovery over 30 minutes, often fail to recognise those around them initially, occasionally aggressive, amnesic for this period, 'wake up' in ambulance or hospital
▪ Recovery: rapid, recognise those around them, embarrassed rather than confused, may vomit, 'wake up' long before paramedics arrive, typically hear before they can see	
▪ Injuries rare, indeed 'red flag' for typical faint	▪ Bitten lateral border of tongue, myalgia for days, rarely shoulder fracture/dislocation; carpet burns suggest non-epileptic attack

2. Benign sensory symptoms and multiple sclerosis

Benign sensory symptoms	Multiple sclerosis
■ Intermittent, periods of normality ■ Often disobey anatomical boundaries, or restricted to specific peripheral nerve ■ No previous neurological symptoms	■ Evolves over few days, persists for days to weeks, then gradually resolves, with no periods of normality ■ Typically spinal cord (ascending bilateral numbness of both legs) or cerebral (hemisensory or arm/leg) ■ May be previous suspicious symptoms, e.g. transient disturbance of vision

3. Benign (primary) headache and sinister (secondary) headache

Benign (primary) headache	Sinister (secondary) headache
■ Present for weeks/months/years; the longer the history, the more likely to be benign (patients think the opposite) ■ Not usually associated with other neurological symptoms ■ Common	■ Short history; beware of thunderclap onset, most will need hospital assessment and CT head ■ Beware of focal or systemic symptoms – neither compatible with most primary headache disorders ■ Even those with above features usually are benign; secondary syndromes all rare by comparison

4. Trigeminal neuralgia and any other facial pain (most commonly idiopathic facial pain)

Trigeminal neuralgia	Any other facial pain (most commonly idiopathic facial pain)
■ Very brief paroxysms of severe jolts of pain ■ Strictly unilateral, affecting cheek/jaw, less commonly eye/frontal region ■ Triggered by talking, eating, wind ■ Often responsive to carbamazepine	■ Usually more persistent dull pain ■ May cross midline, often poorly localised, not obeying anatomical boundaries ■ No specific triggers ■ Often resistant to medication

5. TIA and migrainous aura

TIA	Migrainous aura
■ Short, usually <10 minutes ■ Abrupt onset/offset, little/no evolution ■ Strictly anatomical ■ Negative symptoms (e.g. loss of vision) ■ Usually isolated	■ Typically 10–30 minutes ■ Typically evolves and changes over period ■ Symptoms often cross anatomical borders ■ Positive symptoms (e.g. flashing, fortification spectra) ■ Recurrent, often over long periods

6. Benign memory disturbance and early dementia

Benign memory disturbance	Early dementia
■ Usually younger people (<60 years) ■ Attend alone ■ Subjective symptoms (no one else noted problems) ■ Able to give detailed history ■ Still able to read, follow films/dramas, etc. ■ Considerable variability	■ Older ■ Brought in by relative ■ Patient least aware of problems ■ Often vague, denying problems ■ Often stops activities, as unable to follow ■ May vary but less so

Prescribing Points

1. **Treatment is optional**

   Many neurological disorders require a diagnosis rather than treatment. In other scenarios, most obviously functional symptoms, drugs are best avoided. Always consider the option of no treatment.

2. **Analgesia for headache**

   The natural inclination to escalate analgesia for headaches is rarely successful and usually encourages medication overuse headaches and adverse effects that confuse matters (such as vomiting due to opiates leading to concern about more sinister headaches). Tramadol, co-codamol and similar are not good for anything other than short-term use; NSAIDs are generally a better choice.

3. **Generic versus branded prescribing**

   This is a hot topic for GPs, the NHS and patients. The data are unhelpfully conflicting and so are the relevant advisory bodies. There is no persuasive evidence that there is a meaningful effect in switching brands, but many patients with chronic diseases dislike recurrent brand switching. Recurrent shortages of some drugs (e.g. antiepileptic or PD drugs) are much more of a problem.

4. **Drug titration of CNS active drugs**

   Unsurprisingly, adverse effects of drugs that act on the brain are common, and generally less likely to occur with 'low and slow' titration, often even slower than BNF/manufacturer recommendations.

5. **Measuring blood levels of anti-epileptic drugs**

   In short, don't routinely. The only persuasive indication is to assess whether a patient is actually taking their prescribed drug (non-compliance is a common reason for poor epilepsy control, so always check a level(s) in this scenario, regardless of what compliance the patient reports). Although levels may confirm drug toxicity, this is always a clinical diagnosis, not a number on a blood test.

Anyone on phenytoin or carbamazepine complaining of unsteadiness/ataxia/diplopia is toxic until proven otherwise.

6. **Adherence/compliance/concordance**

   Whichever term one prefers, drugs only have a chance to work if people take them. Thus when dealing with (apparently) treatment-resistant migraine, epilepsy, PD and so on, always consider this possibility. As when patients are reporting alcohol intake, some are parsimonious with the truth when asked, so think of sensitive ways around the topic, how are they coping with their medication, remembering, etc.

7. **Vestibular sedatives**

   These are rarely helpful in the management of long-term 'dizziness' and can prevent recovery. They are ineffective in BPPV (which is cured by the Epley manoeuvre or similar), and long-term prochlorperazine and metoclopramide can be associated with tardive dyskinesias, especially in older people.

8. **Vitamin B$_{12}$**

   B$_{12}$ is a common part of a 'neuro screen' blood battery, and low normal or borderline low results are common. Whilst B$_{12}$ deficiency is well recognised to cause neurological syndromes, such syndromes appear uncommon; much more typical is an incidental result which does not explain the patient's complaint (usually sensory and thus will not respond or resolve with B$_{12}$ replacement). In practice, it is common to see a placebo effect with B$_{12}$ loading, followed by a recurrence of symptoms, leading to requests for more frequent replacement or even repeat loading. Guidelines are often unhelpful in this area, encouraging increasing replacement, and there is much non-scientific 'information' easily found on the internet which causes confusion and distress (similar to arguments over thyroxine replacement). If symptoms fail to resolve with B$_{12}$ replacement, the possibility that B$_{12}$ deficiency was not the cause of the problem should be considered.

OBESITY AND BARIATRIC MEDICINE

Helen Ashby

Ten Pearls of Wisdom

1. View obesity as a chronic disease

It is now widely recognised by multiple medical bodies, including the World Health Organization, that obesity is a chronic disease requiring multiple medical interventions throughout a patient's life. We need to move away from the common misconception that it is a lifestyle problem and instead accept that obesity needs to be given parity with other chronic conditions such as asthma, hypertension and diabetes.

2. Avoid stigma and bias

Weight stigma (social stereotypes and misconceptions about weight and obesity) and weight bias (negative attitudes about obesity and people living with obesity) have significant negative impacts on patients who are trying to lose weight and are sometimes apparent in healthcare practitioners. Patients living with obesity are much more likely to have a chronic disease due to carrying weight, such as cancer, but evidence shows that healthcare practitioners spend less time than average with these patients and are less likely to perform physical examinations on them. There is also evidence to suggest therapeutic inertia – treatments that are not working – are less likely to be changed in patients who carry weight.

3. Ask before addressing weight with a patient, unless they are consulting you about it

If a patient has attended a consultation for another problem, which will be helped by losing weight, a tried-and-tested approach is to ask 'Is it okay to talk about your weight today?' If a patient declines this offer, do not persevere or proceed to give unsolicited advice, however well-meaning. Just state that you are available as and when they might feel ready to talk about it. This is much more likely at least to get the patient thinking about their weight and knowing that they have a receptive healthcare professional when they do wish to discuss it.

 DOI: 10.1201/9781003304586-19

4. Key to successful weight loss is long-term behaviour change

All weight loss interventions are tools to assist weight loss, but the key is long-term behaviour change to reduce calorie intake, which is difficult. Even bariatric surgery has a weight regain phase, usually 3 to 5 years afterwards. Not all patients regain weight, but most do, so surgery should be seen as just one of a number of interventions which may be required to help a patient lose weight and maintain weight loss – behaviour change being the most important. Creating an environment where the patient can address behaviour change may require adequate pain control, good sleep hygiene, a reduction in boredom and help with mental health. Then the patient may feel able to make small but sustained changes to their lifestyle which will have a positive impact on their weight.

5. Losing 5%–10% of initial body weight has huge benefits

A simple reduction of 5%–10% of initial body weight has significant health benefits, even if the patient still has a BMI in the obese range. Weight loss of this degree has consistently been demonstrated to reduce blood pressure, total cholesterol, triglycerides and LDL cholesterol, and improve HDL cholesterol. It improves diabetes control and reduces the progression of impaired glucose tolerance to diabetes. There is also an effect on overall mortality, with all-cause mortality reduced by up to 25%, and even greater reductions in diabetes and cancer-related deaths.

6. The body 'likes' the current weight of the patient

When a patient loses weight, the body increases the amount of 'hunger' hormone (ghrelin) it produces and reduces the 'satisfaction' hormone (leptin) production. Although these are not the only hormonal changes, they have a significant effect and are easy to explain to patients. This leads to patients eating a little more with each portion and being a little less satisfied by their previous portion size. This drip-drip effect of one mouthful more with each meal leads to weight regain after a diet, often to the previous weight and a little more. This is because these hormone changes can last for 12 months after diet and weight loss, and are subtle. Understanding them can help sustain weight loss.

7. Obesity is truly a multisystem disease

Obesity has a significant number of metabolic consequences, which can be physiological or psychological. People living with obesity impact the workload of every healthcare discipline. It is a gateway for cardiovascular disease, diabetes, non-alcoholic fatty liver disease and cancer. Other complications or associations include lung diseases and obstructive sleep apnoea, idiopathic intracranial hypertension, cataracts, pancreatitis and gall bladder disease, gynaecological problems and joint diseases. Addressing long-term lifestyle changes to reduce weight will improve all these problems, and ensure their progression is slowed.

8. Bariatric surgery requires life-long supplementation of vitamins and minerals

Bariatric surgery reduces the size of the stomach and also, in some procedures, bypasses the small intestine where absorption occurs. As a result, these procedures both reduce the volume of food and the surface area available to absorb it. Therefore, twice daily supplementation with a good over-the-counter vitamin and mineral formulation is recommended, as well as supplementation of calcium/vitamin D, together with intramuscular vitamin B_{12} injections every 3 months. The British Obesity and Metabolic Surgery Society (BOMSS) website (https://bomss.org/) has good up-to-date guidelines on post-operative vitamin recommendations.

9. Pregnancy following bariatric surgery requires specialist input

Ideally, female patients should wait at least 12–18 months post-bariatric surgery to fall pregnant. Early pregnancy following bariatric surgery can lead to suboptimal weight loss for the patient. There is also a risk to the baby, especially as it is difficult to ensure adequate nutrition for both patients during the early stages after bariatric surgery. Ideally, Pregnacare multivitamins should be used in the pre-conception phase, with two tablets taken daily; this ensures the correct form of vitamin A is consumed. High-dose folic acid is also recommended to ensure that adequate levels are achieved. Calcium and vitamin D supplements are also required. Careful monitoring of vitamin levels during each trimester is required (there are pregnancy-associated reference ranges) and regular fetal growth monitoring is required. Finally, patients who have had bariatric surgery must not undergo an oral glucose tolerance test, as the high load of sugar will induce hypoglycaemia via dumping syndrome. Therefore, if the patient is at risk of diabetes during pregnancy, monitoring with fasting and post-prandial blood glucose levels for 2 weeks is required to safely assess blood sugar levels. It is recommended that this is done at 16–18 weeks and again at 25–27 weeks.

10. Patients going abroad for weight loss surgery may miss out on pre-assessment and post-operative advice

Because of long waiting lists with the NHS, some patients seek bariatric surgical treatments abroad. These patients may not have had the assessments prior to their surgery that the NHS provides, and can return home without aftercare packages. Whilst some immediate post-operative problems, such as wound infection, can be easily treated, more significant issues do need to be reviewed in secondary care. Longer-term aftercare also needs to be considered. For example, mental health support is key to successful behaviour change to optimise the prospect of long-term success, and patients should be encouraged not to smoke after the operation due to the risk of stomach ulcers at the anastomosis. The BOMSS website offers a good source of information for all clinicians.

Obscure or Overlooked Diagnoses

1. **Acute thiamine deficiency after bariatric surgery**

   In the immediate post-operative period after bariatric surgery, especially over the first 2 weeks, patients who have recurrent vomiting with poor oral intake are at high risk of acute thiamine deficiency. Early symptoms are vague and include poor memory, loss of appetite, fatigue, sleep disturbance and abdominal discomfort. These may all be attributed to the operation and the immediate post-operative phase, so it is easy to overlook this complication. Later symptoms are numbness or pins and needles in extremities and tingling in the legs, which can travel up the body. Immediate treatment with intravenous thiamine is required until tingling and numbness ease, to prevent permanent nerve damage. As symptoms can be vague and difficult to distinguish from post-operative tiredness, a high degree of suspicion is required in patients who have significantly reduced oral intake and persistent vomiting.

2. **Dumping syndrome**

   In the post-operative phase and the longer term, patients are at risk of dumping syndrome. This can occur after all types of bariatric surgery but is more common after a Roux-en-Y bypass. Dumping syndrome occurs when a patient eats (or drinks) something with a high refined sugar content. The early dump occurs 10–30 minutes after a meal; is caused by food and gastric juices entering the small intestine rapidly; and consists of dizziness, cramping abdominal pain, flushing and tachycardia. The late dump occurs 1 to 3 hours after a meal and leads to hypoglycaemia as the body increases the amount of insulin produced to deal with the high sugar load. Patients may complain of the typical symptoms of hypoglycaemia and can feel washed out and tired afterwards, often needing to sleep to recover from the attack. Treatment of dumping syndrome is to identify the trigger foods and to reduce these in the diet. Other medical treatments should be given under specialist supervision.

Easily Confused

1. **Abdominal pain after bariatric surgery**

   About a third of patients after bariatric surgery develop gallstones, usually within the first year. However, there are a couple of other diagnoses that can present with abdominal pain, such as anastomotic ulcers and a rare and difficult-to-diagnose condition called Petersen's hernia. Petersen's hernia is an internal bowel hernia through the mesenteric space. If bariatric surgery was performed many years previously, the defects might not have been sutured, but in modern bariatric surgery, these are all sutured at the time of operation. However, despite this, weight loss can cause these to widen post-operatively. In suspected Petersen's hernia, once other diagnoses have been excluded, a review by a bariatric surgeon is required and possible laparoscopy may be needed to clinch or refute the diagnosis.

Parameter	Anastomotic ulcer	Gallstones	Petersen's hernia
Location of pain	Epigastric	Colicky, central and right upper quadrant	Usually epigastric with dorsal radiation – intermittent in nature
Other symptoms	Nausea, vomiting, reflux	Nausea, vomiting, jaundice	Nausea, vomiting
Relation to food	Worse before food	Worse after eating	Not related to food
Associated risk factors	Smoking	Rapid weight loss	Surgery performed many years ago, significant rapid weight loss after surgery
Dysphagia	Yes	No	Not usually
Investigations	May all be normal, possible anaemia	Abnormal liver function tests (LFTs) in some cases	All normal
Appropriate investigation	Gastroscopy	Ultrasound scan	CT scan/laparoscopy

Prescribing Points

1. **Sustained-release medications**

   After bariatric surgery, gut transit time is decreased, so food and medication travel through the gut much quicker. Therefore, sustained-release medications should be avoided, as they will tend to pass through the gut without being fully absorbed. A typical example is sustained-release metformin, which is commonly prescribed in the cohort who have bariatric surgery.

2. **Weight loss medications**

   At present, there are only three medications that are licensed to help with weight loss. These are orlistat, Saxenda (liraglutide) and Wegovy (semaglutide). No medication will work without dietary changes, and therefore these should be viewed as an adjunct to diet.

   a. *Orlistat*: Orlistat is a lipase inhibitor, which inhibits the absorption of dietary fat. It is used for patients with a BMI of 30 kg/m² or more, or 28 kg/m² if there are risk factors such as type 2 diabetes or hypertension. In a low-fat diet, orlistat helps to remove the fat that cannot be removed from any meal. It tends to give a 50% further reduction in weight over that achieved with diet alone; so if a patient loses a kilogram with dietary changes, they will lose 1.5 kg overall with the addition of orlistat. Orlistat has significant side effects if the patient doesn't adhere to a low-fat diet, and it must be taken 30 minutes before eating. It is contraindicated in chronic malabsorption syndrome and cholestasis, and fat-soluble vitamins should be monitored, as these may not be absorbed satisfactorily.

b. *Liraglutide*: This has strict guidelines concerning prescription. At present, it is available on the NHS for 2 years for patients who fulfil all the following criteria:

- They have a BMI of at least 35 kg/m^2 (or at least 32.5 kg/m^2 for members of minority ethnic groups known to be at equivalent risk of the consequences of obesity at a lower BMI than the white population).
- They have non-diabetic hyperglycaemia (defined as a haemoglobin A1c level of 42 mmol/mol to 47 mmol/mol [6.0% to 6.4%] or a fasting plasma glucose level of 5.5 mmol/L to 6.9 mmol/L).
- They have a high risk of cardiovascular disease based on risk factors such as hypertension and dyslipidaemia.
- It is prescribed in secondary care by a multidisciplinary Tier 3 specialist weight management service.

Weight loss is required to be 5% of initial body weight 12 weeks after the patient is on the maximum dose, and most patients achieve this. The Tier 3 services will ensure achievement of this target in order to continue providing the medication.

c. Semaglutide:

- This is only licensed within specialist weight management services, and the person has at least one weight-related comorbidity and:
    - A BMI of at least 35.0 kg/m^2, or
    - A BMI of 30.0 kg/m^2 to 34.9 kg/m^2 and they meet the criteria for referral to specialist weight management services.
- NICE advises that lower BMI thresholds (usually reduced by 2.5 kg/m^2) should be used for people from South Asian, Chinese, other Asian, Middle Eastern, Black African or African-Caribbean family backgrounds.
- NICE also advises that clinicians should consider stopping semaglutide if less than 5% of the initial weight has been lost after 6 months of treatment.

3. **SGLT2 medications and the liver reduction diet**

When a patient undergoes the liver shrinkage (reduction) diet in the 2 weeks prior to surgery, SGLT2 inhibitors should be stopped 2 to 3 days before the diet is started. The liver reduction diet is an 800 kcal/day diet which all patients undergoing bariatric surgery are asked to adhere to for 2 weeks prior to surgery to ensure the fat is removed from the liver. This allows easy access for safe bariatric surgery. Failure to stop SGLT2 inhibitors can lead to diabetic ketoacidosis, which is potentially life-threatening. Immediately after surgery, due to the very low-calorie intake in the first few days post-operatively, SGLT2 inhibitors should not be recommended and only subsequently restarted on specialist advice.

4. **Hypertension medication regimes may need changing after bariatric surgery**
   Rapid gut transit after bariatric surgery may result in antihypertensive treatment being rapidly absorbed, with its effects wearing off as the day goes on. This can manifest with symptoms of low blood pressure, such as dizziness, in the morning, but then spikes of high blood pressure at the end of the day, which might be noticed on home blood pressure monitoring. As a result, the patient may require their antihypertensive dose to be split into two doses in the day – or, if they are on more than one treatment, these may need to be taken at different times to ensure adequate blood pressure control.

5. **Oral contraceptive pill absorption**
   After bariatric surgery, the oral contraceptive pill may not be absorbed as it was previously. Care must be taken, especially in the immediate post-operative phase, to ensure that adequate contraception is maintained. Solutions include the use of the implant or coil, and should be considered pre-operatively to pre-empt problems.

ONCOLOGY

Karol Sikora

Ten Pearls of Wisdom

1. Beware of persistent symptoms

Any symptom that persists for more than 3 weeks needs careful assessment – particularly if the patient says it's getting progressively worse without any periods of improvement. Headaches, sore throats, lumps, cough, indigestion, vague abdominal pains, changes in bowel habits, bleeding from any orifice, tiredness and unexplained weight loss could all be the first indication of malignancy. Some cancers are notoriously difficult to diagnose, as the symptoms are so vague. Studies have shown that multiple myeloma, ovarian and pancreatic cancer top the list of number of GP visits before hospital referral. If in any doubt, use the cancer pathway. This may well be replaced in the future with a fast-track diagnostic service for all with the creation of a network of Community Diagnostic Hubs.

2. Beware of back pain, incontinence and leg neurology – it could be cord compression

Recognition of this problem in a patient already known to have cancer is suboptimal throughout the system – from the GP through to the emergency room and then the oncology department. Many patients end up spending their last few months in a wheelchair completely unnecessarily, particularly in those tumours where bone metastases are common: lung, prostate and breast. Beware of patients with low-back pain, incontinence, and sensory and motor loss in the legs. Enquire about more subtle changes such as loss of awareness of a full bladder or lack of sensation when passing urine or stool. Don't waste time – call the oncology registrar to avoid long waits. Urgent steroids, palliative radiotherapy or laminectomy can save the day.

3. Take persistent hoarseness seriously

Beware that persistent hoarseness – often without pain or any other symptoms – can be due to cancer in the upper air passages. Refer for an urgent ENT opinion if symptoms are going on for more than 4 weeks, especially if associated with a cough, blood in the saliva and general debility. Often these patients are smokers

---

DOI: 10.1201/9781003304586-20

with COPD, which confuses things. Check for cervical lymphadenopathy and look in the mouth and oropharynx. If you're a dab hand with the mirrors, try to visualise the larynx, but most patients will need a cancer pathway referral for flexible laryngoscopy in the ENT department. First, though, arrange an urgent chest X-ray to ensure the hoarseness is not caused by lung pathology resulting in recurrent laryngeal nerve invasion.

4. Don't take risks with breast lumps

With daily breast cancer stories in the media, many women get worried about cancer – and the worried well can bring the NHS to its knees. But the adage 'no woman should have a lump in the breast' is still valid. We've become very efficient at sorting these problems out nowadays. One-stop breast clinics provide an examination, mammogram, ultrasound, needle biopsy and same-day pathology. They are patient-friendly, with counsellors and specialist nurses. Don't take responsibility for monitoring an undiagnosed breast mass yourself. The days of aspirating supposed breast cysts in the surgery are over – the risk of litigation is high. But you can reassure your patient before you send them for assessment that nine out of ten breast lumps turn out to be benign. There are excellent NICE guidelines on this issue, which in the latest iteration state that all women aged 30 and over with an unexplained breast lump should have a cancer pathway referral.

5. Take vague abdominal pains seriously

These are always difficult to sort out. The cluster of intermittent abdominal pain, tiredness, depression, poor appetite and weight loss is common. Often it is all sorted by a proton pump inhibitor such as lansoprazole and no significant underlying pathology is ever found. But do not be deceived by the apparent clinical improvement that does not last long. Pancreatic, stomach and lower oesophageal cancer can all present in this way. These cancers often take several appointments in the surgery before appropriate investigations are initiated. Refer for an endoscopy and abdominal ultrasound if symptoms persist for more than a month.

6. Ensure men are properly counselled before a PSA test

With increased media awareness and the rise of 'Dr Google', this is a common problem. The PSA is a useful tumour marker for monitoring the progress of prostate cancer and its response to therapy. But it is a useless screening tool, with many false positives.

In the UK, the guidance is to offer the test only when requested, unless it's clinically indicated, with appropriate counselling and preferably written information beforehand. There is simply no evidence that lives are saved by widespread PSA testing in asymptomatic men. Most laboratories give a normal range of 0–4 ng/mL. A pragmatic approach is to reassure men with a value of

4 or less; to repeat after a 4-week interval if levels are from 4 to 10; and if still elevated to refer for a urology opinion, MRI and biopsy. Those with levels above 10 should be referred under the cancer pathway. NICE guidance states that, in symptomatic men, age-specific PSA values should be used to guide whether a 2-week referral is indicated.

7. Be clear on the criteria suggesting possible melanoma – and beware of the subungual version

The 5-year survival of early-stage melanoma is over 90%. But once it spreads to lymph nodes this drops precipitously. Warning signs for urgent referral include a recent change in size, colour or shape of a pigmented lesion. Minor features include a diameter >7 mm, a change in sensation and the presence of inflammation or oozing. Lesions with any of the first three features or three minor ones should be referred urgently to the pigmented lesion clinic. Many offer same-day drop-in appointments where a biopsy can be carried out immediately.

Be particularly careful with the rare but curable subungual melanoma. It usually occurs under the nail of the big toe and looks just like a healing haematoma after trauma. Ask about injury and speed of onset. If no history of trauma and a gradual onset, be particularly suspicious. Easily treated by surgery when localised but not when spread to regional nodes.

8. Constipation alone is unlikely to be a cancer but take day-to-day changes in bowel habits seriously

We all have different bowel patterns related to diet, daily activity and sleep. They tend to be consistent from day to day. The presence of even a small tumour in the sigmoid colon (the most common site for colon cancer) disturbs this normal pattern. This can mean constipation, diarrhoea or just a noticeable irregularity. Constipation alone is unlikely to be cancer-related, but day-to-day changes in bowel habits for more than a month warrant assessment. Blood and mucus can also be present in the stool and most patients seek help promptly for this. Tumours of the caecum may grow to several centimetres before they cause symptoms and can present with anaemia due to blood loss. Any disturbance in bowel habit for over 2 weeks should be followed closely and if persistent a referral for a colonoscopy made.

9. Know the problems caused by cancer treatment

Radiotherapy causes many acute toxicities depending on which part of the body is being irradiated. Reddening of the skin often at the site of the exit dose is common. In upper gastrointestinal and head and neck malignancies, watch for dehydration due to pain on swallowing. Even with marked side effects, it's better not to interrupt a radical course of radiotherapy unless absolutely essential. Ask the patient to speak to the radiographers on the treatment machine and they will advise on the best supportive medications.

With chemotherapy, beware of infection from unusual organisms – this is the most common cause of death during chemotherapy. Any patient with a fever of greater than 38°C for more than an hour and neutropenia as defined by an absolute neutrophil count of less than 0.5×10^9/L requires immediate referral for antibiotics and if necessary, a septic shock protocol. Oncology centres give patients a 24/7 hotline to call – ensure they use it promptly.

10. Second opinions can help patients who have been given a gloomy prognosis

Stopping active cancer treatment and moving to just supportive care to control symptoms is often taken badly by patients and their families. With the media full of breakthrough cancer drugs, people are understandably puzzled why there is nothing for them. Some become angry, while others go into a downward spiral of doom and gloom. Second opinions can help patients with metastatic disease that has become resistant to drugs and hormones. They usually provide reassurance that the correct treatment strategy is in place. Another way of helping is to see if there are any clinical trials they can enter. Cancer Research UK has a useful website with details of active studies: www.cancerresearchuk.org/about-cancer/find -a-clinical-trial.

A sympathetic ear is necessary, emphasising that quality of life rather than longevity is now the main goal. Their local hospice and community palliative care team will prove invaluable with counselling and other supportive care.

Obscure or Overlooked Diagnoses

1. Haematological malignancies

These are fortunately rare but impossible to diagnose without getting a full blood count. The prognosis is very variable and can only be accurate after a suitable laboratory investigation. Avoid getting drawn into outcome conversations until after this is completed and a definitive diagnosis can guide the likely prognosis.

2. Childhood cancers

These are extremely rare and mostly curable. Possible symptoms of something being seriously amiss include lethargy, failure to concentrate, weight loss, difficulty in interacting with others and general withdrawal. It is best to believe the mother if she says something's wrong and it persists. The parents and family will need considerable support during and after what is often protracted chemotherapy and sometimes radiotherapy. However inconvenient, it's worth travelling even a long way to a specialised unit for the best care.

3. **Cancer of unknown primary (CUP)**

This is a very distressing diagnosis for patients as they can't explain to others the type of cancer they actually have. Usually presenting with lymph node, liver or lung metastases, a biopsy may be completely unhelpful in determining the tissue of origin, especially if poorly differentiated. Most cancer centres use a straightforward protocol to try to sort out the best therapy, but the prognosis is generally poor except for lymphomas and germ cell tumours.

4. **Unexplained weight loss**

Unexplained weight loss is a rare presentation of a wide range of different cancers, sometimes with no localising symptoms whatsoever. Get a chest X-ray, abdominal ultrasound and the usual blood work. If no clues become apparent, refer to a local general physician – if you do not have one, then a gastroenterologist is your best bet. Many GPs also have access to urgent assessment via a 'vague symptoms pathway'.

5. **Solitary lymph node enlargement**

The critical diagnostic is a biopsy or excision. The differential is wide: metastasis, lymphoma, inflammation, infection and sarcoid. Avoid jumping to conclusions until the histology is back. With an unexplained cervical node, an ENT referral is probably best in older patients and a general surgeon for those under 60.

Easily Confused

Cancer is a cellular disorder. The only way to clinch the diagnosis is by the histological examination of the removed tissue. A biopsy is the key to sorting out the pairs of benign and malignant conditions listed next. Appropriate specialist referral is necessary as, increasingly, image localisation by CT, MRI or ultrasound is used to ensure the right bit is sampled. The other possible confusion is with infection, especially TB, HIV and a range of exotic tropical illnesses. Always take a travel history. The following are easily and often confused.

1. **Benign and malignant**

Benign	Malignant
■ Benign prostatic hypertrophy	■ Prostate cancer
■ Ductal carcinoma *in situ*	■ Breast cancer
■ Colon adenoma	■ Colon carcinoma
■ Benign brain tumours	■ Gliomas
■ Lobar pneumonia, COPD	■ Lung cancer
■ Benign uterine fibroids	■ Endometrial cancer
■ Keratoacanthoma	■ Basal or squamous skin cancer
■ Congenital cysts on liver and kidney	■ Metastatic deposits

Prescribing Points

As most specialist cancer drugs have to be given in hospital, the most important GP prescribing role concerns supportive care. The 'Palliative care' chapter discusses this.

1. **'Breakthrough' new drugs**

   The internet has driven widespread information about new cancer drugs. Fuelled by press releases from the pharma industry and an excited media, this encourages patients and their relatives to seek out what they perceive as miracle drugs.

   It's very difficult to inject a sense of reality into the hyped-up world of high-cost cancer drugs. We're very good at having the cancer conversation initially, but not so good at telling people there's no more active treatment available. Many patients simply don't hear the message in the clinic and will come to you for help. Second opinions are rarely of real clinical value at this stage but may be the only way to gain acceptance of the situation. You will hear a lot about molecular diagnostics and personalised medicine. The idea is that by using large databases curated by artificial intelligence and the patient's normal and cancer DNA we will be able to optimise their treatment, even for metastatic disease. It's a great idea but, despite the hype, we're not quite there yet. Patients may want to pay for a genomic screen of their cancer to look for 'actionable mutations'. These are specific mutations that may indicate sensitivity to a targeted drug not normally used for their type of cancer. The cost of such a screen varies from £2,000 to £4,000 and takes about 3 weeks depending on the provider. If a suitable drug is found, it may have to be used 'off-label'. This may mean that neither the NHS nor private insurer will pay for it and many new cancer drugs now cost over £10,000 for a month's supply. This all adds to the stress and uncertainty of living with cancer.

2. **Alternative medicine**

   This is a very confusing area. Usually based on anecdotes of great success, many clinics are exploiting vulnerable and susceptible patients who believe their sales pitch. They often charge over £50,000 for a selection of both conventional and unorthodox therapies. Although making a claim to cure cancer and selling such services is illegal in Britain, many patients are going abroad for very dubious treatments. Clinics abound in countries with a less regulated environment including Mexico and Germany. A series of orthodox, often low-dose cancer therapies are mixed with alternatives such as shark's cartilage, laetrile, oxygen therapy and herbal remedies. The evidence base of benefit simply does not exist, but the placebo effect is powerful and of course provides hope. Advise patients to talk to their oncologist. As with financial investments, if it's too good to be true, it probably is. Complementary therapies such as massage, reflexology, acupuncture and reiki are popular and widely offered by palliative care teams. There is evidence that they can improve quality of life but not longevity.

OPHTHALMOLOGY

Omar Rafiq

Ten Pearls of Wisdom

1. **Consider the diagnosis of chalazion in apparent recurrent styes**
   Chalazia and styes are different things. Chalazia occur because of a blocked
   meibomian gland. They are not usually painful unless infected. Styes, on the
   other hand, are infected hair follicles on the lid margin. They present with a
   painful yellow lesion around the lid margin. Styes are usually self-limiting,
   resolving within 1 or 2 weeks – this can be accelerated by warm compresses.
   Occasionally they may require antibiotics. An infected chalazion can resemble a
   stye, so consider this possibility in 'recurrent styes'.

2. **Blepharitis is common and causes a huge variety of symptoms**
   Blepharitis causes inflammation of the eyelids and can result in a multitude of
   symptoms, including a foreign body or burning sensation, excessive tearing,
   itching, photophobia, red and swollen eyelids, redness of the eye, blurred vision,
   frothy tears, dry eye or crusting of the eyelashes on awakening. Examination may
   reveal crusty red eyelids and a lash margin with debris stuck to it. The eyes may
   be mildly red and there may be 'frothy' secretions at the lid margin. Treat with
   lid hygiene. A typical regime is a warm compress, followed by a cleansing of the
   lashes from the roots, aiming to clear the debris, using cotton gauze softened
   with lukewarm water (advise patients to keep their eyes closed while doing this
   so as not to cause corneal injury). Blepharitis rarely resolves, so patients need to
   continue these measures indefinitely. Severe blepharitis might need a short course
   of antibiotics and topical steroids.

3. **Beware of sticky eyes or conjunctivitis within the first 28 days
   of birth**
   Babies don't usually produce tears for the first 6 to 8 weeks of life. So sticky
   eyes or conjunctivitis within the first month should be viewed as ophthalmia
   neonatorum and referred to paediatrics for appropriate management. A watery
   eye in a child, on the other hand, is quite common – once babies start producing
   tears, then a blocked nasolacrimal duct can become evident. This duct widens
   as the child grows, so about 90% resolve within the first year. Parents can be

DOI: 10.1201/9781003304586-21

advised on lacrimal massage – compression of the tear sac forces fluid through the nasolacrimal duct, causing the obstruction to open by hydraulic pressure.

4. Remember temporal arteritis when elderly patients present with acute visual disturbance

Always consider this diagnosis in elderly patients who have painless visual loss that can be very sudden. Patients may complain of intermittent or even complete loss of vision or flashes/flickering of lights. There may be temporal pain or tenderness, and features of polymyalgia may also be present. Jaw claudication may develop after chewing for some time; immediate pain on chewing is usually temporomandibular dysfunction. Temporal arteritis typically occurs in people over the age of 50. If visual symptoms are present, patients should be referred to ophthalmology urgently, as the risk of blindness is significant. If there are no visual symptoms, then patients are usually referred to rheumatology. As long as there are no contraindications, it may be prudent to commence oral steroids at 40–60 mg daily if it is felt there will be a delay in diagnosis, specifically in the patient undergoing a temporal artery biopsy. Starting steroids within the first day or so of symptoms can drastically reduce the disease burden, however, a delay of 48–72 hours or more in treatment can cause irreversible damage. A temporal artery biopsy can still be performed and provide valuable information a few weeks after the initiation of steroid treatment. It is worth also considering prophylactic treatment for gastrointestinal protection with a proton pump inhibitor and bisphosphonate/calcium/vitamin D for bone protection for patients on steroid therapy.

5. The presence of a cataract does not automatically imply a need for surgery

Cataracts should be viewed as part of a spectrum rather than a fixed entity. Some patients can have a very little cataract but suffer significant visual symptoms. Similarly, even with a significant cataract, a patient may perceive no real issues. Vision does not just comprise reading letters from a chart but also involves other important factors, such as contrast sensitivity and brightness. Informing patients of the risks and benefits of surgical intervention allows a patient to make an informed choice as to whether surgery is warranted at that particular time, depending on the degree of disability the symptoms are causing.

6. Monocular diplopia is usually due to an eye problem, whereas binocular diplopia is usually neurological

Assessing whether diplopia is monocular or binocular is straightforward. Monocular diplopia is double vision in one eye that persists when the other eye is covered. This is rarer than binocular diplopia, which resolves when either eye is covered. Monocular causes include astigmatism, cataract, dry eye and macular degeneration. Binocular diplopia can result from a squint, multiple sclerosis, myasthenia gravis and thyroid eye disease.

7. Assessing vision doesn't necessarily require a Snellen chart

Away from the hospital setting, not every organisation has a Snellen chart. But a good discriminator that gives a reasonable idea about vision simply involves asking the patient if their vision seems reduced. Also, you can use different sizes of fonts – for example, in a newspaper – at a distance of 1 metre to see if there is a difference between the two eyes. If the vision is very poor, you can proceed to checking if the patient can see how many fingers you are holding up, your hand moving or a light source – in that order. Also, nowadays, there are lots of apps that you can download onto your smartphone that provide a Snellen chart, colour vision chart and so on, which can prove very useful.

8. Pay close attention when somebody insists they feel something in their eye – they are usually right

Listen to the history – it will give you big clues. What were they doing? Was there a gust of wind that blew something in their eye? Were they doing woodwork or drilling without safety glasses on? Have they been gardening? The history will probably give you a cause-and-effect scenario. If the patient is very uncomfortable, try instilling topical anaesthetic drops to ease examination. Look carefully in the inferior fornix by asking the patient to look up and then also superotemporally and superonasally. Often, the foreign body will have embedded under the superior lid, so it is important to try to gently evert this lid. This can easily be done by pulling the upper lid down (gently holding the eyelashes/lid margin) and using a cotton bud to evert the lid back on itself. If a foreign body is evident, use a cotton bud to remove it if possible. Do ask the patient to look down and also inferonasally and inferotemporally, as the superior fornix is deep – foreign bodies can lurk away from view. If the eye is numb, another tip is to use the cotton bud tip to gently massage the conjunctiva downwards to see if anything can be 'coaxed' down into view. I can recall a full rose thorn being dislodged this way even though on initial inspection nothing was visible on everting the upper lid. If you have access to fluorescein drops or strips, these are worth using – many pen torches have a blue filter that highlights any corneal abrasion. Patients with a corneal abrasion may not have a foreign body in the eye, but the abrasion itself will cause pain and the 'sensation' of something in the eye. As long as a thorough examination is carried out to exclude a foreign body, the symptoms should disappear when the abrasion is treated.

9. Beware of the contact lens wearer with a red eye

Have a very low threshold to refer these patients to ophthalmology. Unfortunately, contact lens hygiene advice is not always made clear. Contact lens cases should be kept clean, with the appropriate contact lens solution used to disinfect the lenses. Patients should be advised not to swim, shower or sleep with their lenses in (some lenses are manufactured to be kept in but the risk of an infection increases). Water contains parasites, and if patients expose themselves to such risks, they can develop sight-threatening infections.

10. **Uveitis patients tend to know they are having a flare-up**

They may feel an 'aura' or symptoms a few days before clinical signs show. So you may not necessarily see a red photophobic eye when they initially present – don't wait for it to develop before starting treatment. They will invariably seek help early and tend to volunteer 'this is my uveitis flaring up'. It is wise to commence topical steroid drops early in these patients to prevent a full-blown uveitis flare-up. In most hospital eye clinics, patients with recurrent uveitis are given an open appointment or are on a PIFU (patient-initiated follow-up) pathway.

Obscure or Overlooked Diagnoses

1. **Ocular migraines**

These can give rise to visual loss that can last from a few minutes to half an hour. They can cause blurring of vision, partial vision loss, scotomas and flashes of light, and can be associated with a headache. The ocular aura is usually unilateral and the photopsias are typically described as 'multicoloured speckles' of light similar to looking through a kaleidoscope. They should, however, be a diagnosis of exclusion and need to be distinguished from other entities such as amaurosis fugax or retinal detachment – especially when patients do not have a history of migraine, are over the age of 50 and have other medical conditions.

2. **Molluscum contagiosum of the eyelids**

This is common in children and results in small umbilicated nodules along the lid margin. These can shed viral particles causing chronic follicular conjunctivitis, which is usually unilateral. It does not need treating unless it is a problem – in which case, the lesions can be frozen with cryotherapy, scraped off or treated with topical agents. There should be a balance struck between leaving alone and treating, as the treatment itself can cause scarring, so patients should be counselled appropriately, given that the condition usually disappears spontaneously after a few months.

3. **Floppy eyelid syndrome**

Floppy eyelid syndrome usually affects middle-aged, overweight males and presents with unilateral or bilateral chronic papillary conjunctivitis. The eyelids are lax and floppy with a large fornix. It can cause ocular irritation and discharge. The syndrome is associated with sleep apnoea. Surgical correction is possible if the symptoms are severe.

4. **Recurrent erosion syndrome**

   Individuals may have a history of a prior corneal injury recently or even many years back, though they may have to think hard to remember it. Typically, patients wake up and, as they open their eyes, the corneal epithelium 'sloughs' off. As the cornea is heavily innervated, the result is severe pain and a foreign body sensation. The treatment is topical antibiotics and lubricants. If it persists, consider referring to ophthalmology, as phototherapeutic keratectomy (PTK) laser can help strengthen the corneal bonds. Patching the eye for 24–48 hours with a cotton eye patch/gauze/dressing is a very simple but effective pain-control method, as is the use of dilating agents such as cyclopentolate drops, twice a day for 2 or 3 days (although the pain tends to subside greatly after the first 24 hours or so with the initiation of treatment; if so the dilating drops can be stopped).

5. **Thyroid eye disease (TED)**

   In this condition, the eye muscles and surrounding fatty tissue swell, causing the eye to bulge forward – 'proptosis'. If the eye protrudes too much, the small amount of 'slack' that the optic nerve has is reduced, compromising the nerve and causing loss of vision. TED can also cause exposure keratopathy. It needs to be recognised and promptly treated to avoid blindness. An easy way to check for proptosis is to look from above and behind the patient to see if the eyes protrude. Another sign is evidence of any scleral 'show', that is, any sclera showing from the lower lid margin to the cornea – normally there is none. It is also prudent to check for extraocular muscle movements; some patients have restricted eye movements, especially looking up. Approximately 25% of people with Graves' disease develop TED. Although many patients with TED have abnormal thyroid hormone levels, some have symptoms in the absence of clinical or biochemical markers. Mild cases can be managed with lubricating eye drops, whereas severe cases may need immunosuppression and decompression surgery. Smoking worsens TED, so patients should strongly be encouraged to stop.

Easily Confused

1. **Conjunctivitis and blocked nasolacrimal duct obstruction (NLDO) in a baby**

Conjunctivitis	NLDO
▪ Acute	▪ Presents after 5 to 6 weeks of age as tears start to be produced
▪ Global discharge	
▪ Mild/moderate photophobia	▪ Discharge elicited over the NLD area
▪ Mild irritation/discomfort	▪ No photophobia
▪ Global conjunctival redness/chemosis	▪ No pain/obvious discomfort (unless infected)
	▪ No conjunctival redness

2. Ocular migraine and retinal detachment

Ocular migraine	Retinal detachment
■ Multicoloured speckles/flickers of light	■ Flash 'arc' of light
■ Lights usually start centrally	■ Lights normally peripheral
■ Can be associated with headache	■ No headache
■ No floaters	■ Sudden onset floaters/flashes of lights
■ Visual loss, if any, usually lasts less than half an hour	■ Progressive field loss

3. Acute glaucoma and chronic open-angle glaucoma

Acute glaucoma	Chronic open-angle glaucoma
■ Acute painful eye	■ No pain
■ Red eye	■ No red eye (unless drop allergy)
■ Intraocular pressure very high	■ Intraocular pressure raised but not high enough to be causing pain
■ Very tense orbit	■ No tense orbit
■ Nausea and vomiting	■ No associated nausea or vomiting
■ Small eyes (hypermetropes)	■ Usually in normal/large eyes (myopes)
■ Decreased vision	■ Usually have good central vision
■ Mid-dilated sluggish pupil	■ Normal-reacting pupil

4. Conjunctivitis and acute anterior uveitis

Conjunctivitis	Acute anterior uveitis
■ Discharge	■ No discharge (though may water)
■ Uni-/bilateral	■ Usually unilateral
■ Usually gross conjunctival injection	■ May get minimal conjunctival injection, possibly subtle just around corneal edge ('ciliary flush')
■ May need topical antibiotics	■ Needs topical steroids

5. Episcleritis and scleritis

Episcleritis	Scleritis
■ Inflammation of superficial episclera	■ Inflammation involving the sclera
■ Common	■ Uncommon
■ No pain usually	■ Painful – especially moving eye
■ Self-limiting	■ Usually needs systemic treatment
■ Not sight-threatening	■ Sight-threatening

Prescribing Points

1. **Avoid indiscriminate prescribing – especially topical steroids**
   If you are not sure of the diagnosis, avoid topical medications and, in particular, steer clear of steroids (unless a confirmed case of recurrent/chronic uveitis as described earlier); if the patient has herpes simplex keratitis, for example, this can exacerbate the situation. It is wise to be prudent; in a case of suspected conjunctivitis that is not resolving with standard treatment, ophthalmic referral is recommended.

2. **Check on compliance**
   A common cause of apparent treatment failure is poor compliance or problems administering drops. Check this before changing the treatment regime. Ideally, anticipate problems – if the patient has very bad hand arthritis, instilling drops will inevitably be difficult. Ascertain if other family members or friends can instil the drops; it may be necessary to arrange district nurse assistance for a short period.

3. **Avoid unnecessary medication changes in chronic glaucoma patients**
   A patient whose condition is well controlled should not have their medication changed unnecessarily from one manufacturing company to the next. This only induces anxiety for the patient and, although it may contain the same medication, the excipients can be very different and can cause allergic eye disease and discomfort. This is especially the case if patients have been on preservative-free medication and are then converted to a preserved option (usually out-of-cost considerations). Preservatives contribute massively to red eyes.

ORTHOPAEDICS

Phil Clelland and John Leach

Ten Pearls of Wisdom

1. Cauda equina syndrome can evolve slowly and may be incomplete

The commonest cause is compression of the cauda equina by a prolapsed intervertebral disc. Traditionally we are taught to enquire about urinary incontinence, and to seek perineal sensory changes and reduced anal sphincter tone. But physical signs are unreliable, and by the time the patient presents with incontinence, the situation is likely to be irretrievable. So nuanced history-taking is required. Reduced awareness of bladder filling, loss of the urge to void and decreased sensation when passing urine may be significant, and referral should be made on suspicion. You may well end up referring more patients, but you are less likely to miss a case. The patient requires urgent imaging (usually an MRI scan) with a view to neurosurgical decompression.

2. Don't forget to check for scoliosis in children – and refer if detected

Although mild disease may be painless, check for scoliosis in children and adolescents with back pain. The most common form is adolescent idiopathic scoliosis (80%–85%). Use the Adam's forward bend test: look for a unilateral hump when the patient bends forward so the spine is horizontal. Some cases just require observation, although presentation under the age of 12 and female sex signify an increased risk for curve progression. But in reality, the GP is likely to refer all for initial assessment. The scoliosis can be functional, caused by a leg length discrepancy. This is identified by sitting the patient down – if the curve disappears on sitting, leg length discrepancy is the culprit. This too requires orthopaedic referral, for consideration of equalisation.

3. The majority of disc prolapse symptoms resolve spontaneously – but consider early referral if there is lower limb neurology

About 70%–80% of intervertebral disc prolapses resolve within 12 months. The amount of pain and the chance of resolution don't correlate well with the size of disc herniation. The pain generators in a disc prolapse are the chemicals

DOI: 10.1201/9781003304586-22

released around the nerve, not the physical compression. The latter is, however, responsible for the neurological deficit. Early surgical decompression probably does have better outcomes. This guides the rationale for investigation and referral of back pain: focal lower limb neurology should have an MRI scan and neurosurgical referral if the patient is amenable to surgery. In the absence of neurology, the mainstay of treatment is analgesia and physiotherapy.

4. Elbow pain is not always tennis elbow – but it if is, avoid steroid injections

The history is the key. A sudden onset or deterioration may indicate a lateral epicondyle tendon tear rather than classical tennis elbow, which usually has a more insidious onset. This is important because tears – which can be demonstrated on MRI – require surgical repair to improve symptoms. Steroid injections should not be used for tennis elbow because of the adverse risk–benefit profile. Nonsteroidal anti-inflammatory drugs (NSAIDs) are useful alongside physiotherapy. Newer treatment strategies include platelet-rich plasma injections under ultrasound guidance. This needs to be coupled with an initial short period of rest followed by eccentric exercises targeted at the wrist extensors.

5. Beware bruising after shoulder trauma

Bruising after a shoulder injury should be taken very seriously. It signifies either a fracture or a significant tendon/ligament injury – these patients need to be referred for an X-ray immediately.

In a young adult in this situation, a normal X-ray suggests serious soft tissue damage. The patient should be assessed in an upper limb fracture clinic or in an urgent outpatient appointment. Early repair of acute, large, non-degenerative rotator cuff tears have significantly better outcomes because it avoids the complications of muscle retraction and atrophy. Bear in mind, too, that trauma does not cause an acute frozen shoulder. X-ray is mandatory to rule out fracture and/or dislocation.

6. 'Pain plus misery' are the indicators for total joint arthroplasty

When you hear this combination of complaints, it's probably time for a major joint replacement. So ask your patients to put up with the pain as long as they can – using analgesia and the usual conservative measures – but when the pain becomes 'misery', an arthroplasty is likely to be of benefit. It is important to advise these patients to lose weight if appropriate and to give up smoking. Smoking significantly increases the risk of deep infection ($\times 2.4$) and implant revision ($\times 1.8$) following hip or knee arthroplasty. These statistics may well help motivate them to quit.

7. 'Urgent' knees are those that lock or swell rapidly after trauma

A locked knee in flexion suggests a meniscal 'bucket handle tear' requiring same-day referral – early repair can prevent future osteoarthritis. Rapid post-traumatic swelling – onset within an hour or so of injury – represents intra-articular bleeding caused by an ACL injury, fracture or patella dislocation. This needs an urgent X-ray to rule out a fracture, then referral to be seen within 2 weeks. Slow-onset swelling developing over an evening or the next day is usually caused by a meniscal tear, articular cartilage injury or exacerbation of pre-existing osteoarthritis. Urgent referral is not required unless there is locking. Watchful waiting is reasonable with subsequent routine referral biased towards younger, active patients with disabling symptoms.

8. Redness within the first few post-operative days is likely to be post-traumatic bruising rather than infection

True infection takes a week or so to manifest. It causes redness around the wound, increasing pain and restriction of movement. Late stages are wound discharge and systemic symptoms such as fever. If the patient is systemically unwell, admit urgently. Ideally, speak to the surgical team before starting empiric antibiotics. Post-operative sutures sometimes cause concern. If they are white or clear, they will be dissolvable, whereas coloured sutures can be dissolvable but may need to be removed.

9. A straight leg raise (SLR) can identify quad, knee and hip pathology as well as lumbosacral radiculopathy

The SLR commonly identifies lumbosacral radiculopathy (sciatica). A positive test comprises pain radiating down the back of the leg when it's passively raised between 30° and 70°. The SLR is also helpful in various knee extensor mechanism injuries: quadriceps tendon rupture, patella fracture and patellar tendon rupture, which all present with pain and an inability to actively straight leg raise. Management should include knee immobilisation to prevent tendon retraction and fracture clinic assessment for possible surgery. Hip fractures do not always present classically and may not be visible on X-rays. The inability to actively straight leg raise, groin pain and limited hip rotation in combination help identify these occult hip fractures.

10. Beware the unresolving 'ankle sprain'

An underdiagnosed injury is the high ankle or syndesmotic sprain – damage to the ligamentous complex between the distal tibia and fibula. Suspect this when the mechanism of injury includes ankle rotation. Signs include toe walking to avoid painful dorsiflexion, pain with combined passive ankle dorsiflexion, and external rotation and syndesmotic pain provoked by compressing the tibia and fibula at mid-calf. Once the diagnosis is suspected, patients should be non-weight-bearing and seen in fracture clinic. Bear in mind, too, that patients with a 'weak' ankle following injury or recurrent sprains may be suffering chronic ligament injury or have 'functional instability' caused by painful scar impingement within the ankle joint. Physiotherapy or arthroscopy may be required.

Obscure and Overlooked Diagnoses

1. **Calcific tendinitis**
   In the absence of trauma, sudden incapacitating shoulder pain may well be
   calcific tendinitis. The patient is often in agony with disturbed sleep. An X-ray
   will reveal calcification in the rotator cuff. Treatment consists initially of an
   ultrasound-guided steroid injection into the calcific deposit.

2. **Ulnar nerve problems**
   The ulnar nerve can be trapped at the elbow (cubital tunnel syndrome) or
   the wrist (Guyon's canal compression). Numbness on the dorsal and volar
   ulnar side of the hand suggests compression at the elbow, while numbness
   only on the volar side suggests compression in Guyon's canal. Urgent referral
   is required if the patient has motor features. Early motor symptoms involve
   the hand feeling clumsy due to weakness in the intrinsic muscles – affecting
   intricate activities such as doing up buttons or shoe laces, writing and picking
   up fine objects. Late signs, such as muscle wasting, may be irreversible, so refer
   early.

3. **Popeye biceps rupture**
   Popeye biceps sign with pain and bruising distally on the front of the elbow
   may indicate a distal biceps rupture. Repair should ideally be performed within
   10–14 days. The biceps is the main forearm supinator, so this movement will
   be most affected. Popeye sign with tenderness at the front of the shoulder is a
   proximal long head of biceps rupture – not an urgent referral. Often, surgery
   is not needed as this injury tends to occur in older patients and causes fewer
   problems.

4. **Missed scaphoid fracture**
   A goalkeeper blocking a shot is a common mechanism for scaphoid fracture and
   should always be taken seriously when presenting with wrist pain. Look out for a
   restricted range of movement, especially extension, with pain and swelling in the
   anatomical snuffbox plus pain on telescoping the thumb.

5. **Iliotibial band syndrome**
   This condition often affects runners, causing pain in the lateral aspect of the
   knee. It is caused by inflammation of the iliotibial band, which connects the iliac
   crest of the pelvis to the lateral proximal tibia. The iliotibial band rubs over the
   lateral femoral condyle at the knee during flexion and extension, causing pain.
   This is often well localised but can radiate up the lateral aspect of the thigh.
   Treatment usually involves activity modification and physiotherapy.

Easily Confused

1. Spinal claudication and vascular claudication

Spinal claudication	Vascular claudication
Pain relieved by sitting	Pain relieved by standing, sitting or stopping walking
Pain starts proximally and goes down the legs	Pain starts in the calves and moves up the legs
Pain less severe walking uphill	Pain more severe walking uphill
Pulses present	Pulses absent

2. Shoulder osteoarthritis (OA) and shoulder impingement and frozen shoulder

Shoulder OA	Shoulder impingement	Frozen shoulder
Pain deep inside the shoulder	Pain in the badge area	Pain is global
Poor external rotation with the arm at the side and the elbow bent *with* crepitus	Normal external rotation	Poor external rotation with the arm at the side and the elbow bent *without* crepitus
Often not able to get shoulder to the impingement position	Shoulder pain with impingement test: arm is internally rotated while abducted to 90 degrees	Place your hand on the top of the shoulder to fix the scapula – no abduction is possible
X-ray shows reduction in joint space, osteophytes, cysts and possible proximal migration of humeral head	X-ray normal	X-ray normal

3. Carpal tunnel syndrome and cervical nerve root pain

Carpal tunnel syndrome	Cervical nerve root pain
Pins and needles at night with 'wake and shake'	No nocturnal symptoms
Symptoms – usually pins and needles – in the thumb index and middle fingers	Symptoms – usually pain – in any finger, depending on nerve root affected
Upper limb reflexes normal	Upper limb reflexes reduced or absent, e.g. loss of triceps reflex for C7
Neck and arm movements do not alter symptoms	Neck extension makes arm pain worse; neck flexion may improve the pain Arm above the head may ease the pain
Axial load on the head in lateral tilt makes no difference	Axial compression of the head in lateral tilt to the affected side makes the pain worse (Spurling's test)

4. Thumb OA and de Quervain's tenosynovitis

Thumb OA	De Quervain's tenosynovitis
Usually over 50	Any age
Not related to pregnancy	Often related to pregnancy or unaccustomed repeated lifting of a young child
Thumb base may looked squared off	Swelling more proximal to the radial styloid
Pain well localised to the dorsal thumb carpometacarpal (CMC) joint	Pain along the line of the thumb and radial border of the wrist
Pain worse with thumb pinch, especially with rotation, such as a key in the door	Pain worse with flexion of the thumb into the palm, especially with ulnar deviation

5. Septic joint effusion and aseptic joint effusion

Septic joint effusion	Aseptic joint effusion
Rapid onset over a few hours progressively getting more painful hour on hour	Slower onset over a day or two and not excessively painful
Redness and warmth	No temperature nor colour change
Unable to weight-bear or move the joint without agony	Able to weight-bear and move the joint although may feel stiff and achy
Systemic features	Systemically well

Prescribing Points

1. **Topical and oral NSAIDs**
   Consider using topical NSAIDs as an alternative to oral NSAIDs in osteoarthritis. Suitable patients include those with mild-moderate pain and those intolerant of oral NSAIDs. However, the benefits of topical NSAIDs may not be sustained for more than a few months. Offer a topical NSAID to people with knee osteoarthritis, and consider it for people with osteoarthritis that affects other joints. Topical NSAIDs are superior to placebo in achieving significant pain reduction, have low numbers needed to treat and have a similar GI risk profile to placebo. The most common adverse effect is a mild, local skin reaction. This may be related to the 'vehicle' used, so a trial of an alternative is recommended in this situation.

2. **Steroids for joint injections**
   Intra-articular steroid injections can be a useful option to manage pain and improve function in osteoarthritic joints. They are most commonly used in the shoulder, first carpometacarpal joint, hip, knee and ankle. Response is highly

variable and is often short-lived. The general consensus among surgeons for the maximum number of injections for a single joint is three per year. Many won't perform arthroplasty within 3 months of a steroid injection into that joint due to infection risk.

3. **Medication for low back pain and sciatica**

For pain in either scenario, current guidance advises drug treatments for symptom relief such as NSAIDs, or, as second line, the short-term use of codeine with or without paracetamol. We should avoid gabapentinoids, other antiepileptics and benzodiazepines for managing sciatica – there is no overall evidence of benefit and these drugs can, of course, be harmful. Also, avoid opioids for chronic sciatica. In patients already taking any of these drugs for sciatica, discuss the risks involved and come to a joint decision about whether to stop them, acknowledging the problems associated with withdrawal.

PAEDIATRICS

Peter Heinz

Ten Pearls of Wisdom

1. **All infants regurgitate feeds, but not all have gastro-oesophageal reflux disease**
   Regurgitating feeds is something every infant experiences. Some infants try to re-swallow what has just washed up, often leading to impressive periods of breath holding and gulping, described by worried parents as 'choking'. Thankfully, babies are designed to deal with this problem, and to my knowledge, there has never been a baby death attributable to reflux. When associated with pain, faltering growth or feeding refusal, this normal phenomenon of reflux becomes gastro-oesophageal reflux disease. Only then should treatment be considered.

2. **Colic: It is just a phase**
   Colic is a recognised medical condition, listed in the Rome III criteria for functional gastrointestinal disorders. What is lacking, though, is a true understanding of what colic actually is and – most important – how to deal with it. Where it becomes complicated is when trying to differentiate it from similar elusive diagnoses such as gastro-oesophageal reflux disease, milk protein allergy and 'purple crying' episodes. What we do know is that it does settle on its own with no proven long-term ill health effects, colic treatments do not work and the parents rather than the baby require all our support.

3. **Healthy babies may scream until they are purple in the face**
   Recurrent episodes of screaming without obvious reason in otherwise healthy babies pose a significant burden – to their parents and families, but also to the health economy due to frequent attendance and inappropriate secondary care referrals resulting in overinvestigation and unnecessary treatments. To clarify: I am referring to the type of screaming that will leave your ears ringing long after the family has left your consultation room! A thriving child without feeding difficulties that examines normally requires only parental reassurance, health visitor involvement and signposting to online resources.

DOI: 10.1201/9781003304586-23

4. Know when to worry about rashes

The key issue when dealing with rashes is to establish whether the child is well (if unwell, consider meningococcal septicaemia, anaphylaxis and leukaemia). If the child is well, you may then consider whether the rash is specific, which implies potential management options, or non-specific, when it is likely to resolve over time under your observant gaze.

5. Parents are often wrong when suspecting food allergy …

All sorts of paediatric ills, especially if recurrent with variable skin, respiratory or gut symptoms, will at some point trigger the inevitable question: 'Doctor, could this be an allergy?' In the vast majority of cases, the answer is a resounding no! Allergic reactions are trigger- and threshold-dependent and easily identified by the family keeping a symptom diary focusing on reactions within minutes or a few hours, even in infants that are suspected to have a non-IgE–mediated milk allergy. Referral for allergy testing is only the next step in confirming the diagnosis, not a screening test.

6. … But parents have a fine-tuned sense when it comes to developmental abnormalities

Developmental milestones in normal children vary greatly and significant pathology often leads to more than one category (gross motor, fine motor, vision, hearing and speech, and social) being affected. If the parents are not concerned, there is probably nothing wrong with the child – whereas, if they are, you probably should be, too.

7. Diagnosing milk allergy in infants is a matter of trial and error

Excessive screaming, faltering growth, blood in the stool, vomiting and severe eczema are among many symptoms attributed to possible milk allergy and because these are common and non-specific, establishing a clear link can be challenging. In the majority of infants in the pre-weaning age, milk 'allergy' is non-IgE–mediated and hence not detectable on conventional allergy testing (thankfully, the management remains the same). The only route to diagnosis is a switch to an extensively hydrolysed formula for no longer than 2 weeks and then – this is important – a re-challenge with a normal formula or breast milk. In breastfed babies, mothers will need to embark on a strict dairy-free diet. Lactose-free formulae are not indicated unless the child has profuse, green diarrhoea with every feed as the only symptom and a triggering diarrhoeal illness. Involvement of a dietitian becomes a necessity at the latest from 6 months of age onwards to support dairy-free weaning.

8. A breastfed baby with faltering growth needs calories, not a paediatrician

Exclusively breastfed infants are often referred for a paediatric opinion because of faltering growth. Typically, these infants are 'feeding all the time' but demonstrate static growth. The clinical assessment would be expected to show an infant that is alert, pink, with no respiratory symptoms such as fast breathing and normal cardiac auscultation. No laboratory tests are required and an increase in calorie supply is the sole priority. This may be via intensified breastfeeding support and/or supplementation of feeds with formula/expressed breast milk. If your intervention is successful, you should expect to see an effect on the weight gain within 1 week at most.

9. Asymmetrical hip creases alone do not need imaging

Many clinicians do seem to believe that asymmetrical skin creases of the thigh require hip imaging. Of course, the reality is a little less simplistic but reassuringly straightforward. For children who have started walking with a normal gait, do not worry (the more obsessive among us may also confirm equal leg length, easily measured in primary care). If the child is not walking yet but the hips examine normally and leg length is normal, again, don't worry and simply observe gross motor development. If you have further clinical concerns such as leg length difference, walking with a limp or delayed milestones, the most appropriate investigation would be a hip X-ray from a weight of more than 8 to 10 kg on (equivalent to roughly 6 to 8 months of age) because ultrasound does not work reliably beyond this threshold.

10. Preschoolers: Not everything that wheezes is asthma

The underlying causes of preschool wheeze are multiple, and long-term outcome predictions are difficult. To complicate matters, 'wheeze' is a commonly used term for a number of respiratory noises, and confirmation of the presence of bronchospasm, such as high-pitched expiratory noise, prolonged expiratory phase and chest hyperinflation or deformity, is important. For practical purposes, it makes sense to categorise wheezy children into having either 'episodic viral wheeze' (EVW) or 'multiple trigger wheeze' (MTW). Children with MTW resemble an adult asthma phenotype, with symptoms on most days, triggered not only by viral infections but also by exercise, smoke and allergens. In contrast, EVW only occurs with clear evidence of an upper respiratory tract infection (URTI) and causes no interval symptoms. While children with MTW are most at risk of undertreatment, the opposite is probably true of children with viral-induced wheeze (VIW). In terms of managing preschool wheeze, one is well advised to check the BTS (British Thoracic Society) guidance regularly, as recommendations are evolving frequently.

Obscure or Overlooked Diagnoses

1. Teething

Parents attribute various symptoms to teething, including irritability, decreased feeding and fever – even when their children have no evidence of dental eruption. While there is some evidence linking such non-specific symptoms (including a low-grade fever) with teething, expert views on the strength of the association vary. Health professionals, therefore, need to be cautious when blaming a young child's fever and irritability merely on teething, and safety-net carefully.

2. **Breath holding**

Upset, fear or pain may trigger a child to stop breathing and lose consciousness for a few seconds, occasionally with brief, seizure-like twitching. Some people distinguish between blue spells and white spells, but the underlying mechanism, a brief period of asystole, is the same. These episodes, correctly termed 'reflex anoxic seizures/syncope', may occur as early as with the first immunisations and peak in early childhood. Iron deficiency anaemia can be a contributory factor. Every case should also have a baseline ECG to rule out long QT syndrome – otherwise, reassurance is in order.

3. **Growing pains**

Typically, the child wakes at least once per night, often at a similar time, with throbbing pain in the lower legs that improves on rubbing and settles within an hour. Analgesia may not help. The pain occurs exclusively at night and can occur in clusters. The child is fine in the morning, often with no recollection of the previous night's events. This contrasts with the behaviour of children with bone pain due to a tumour, an undiagnosed fracture or subacute osteomyelitis. The underlying mechanism is elusive, although children with a degree of joint hypermobility appear to be particularly susceptible.

4. **Tongue-tie (ankyloglossia)**

This is a relatively common congenital anomaly (or normal variation, depending on your viewpoint), present in 4% to 10% of infants. Diagnosis, clinical significance and management are controversial. There is no evidence to suggest tongue-tie causes speech problems in later life nor that any speech problems that might occur are prevented by early infancy frenotomy.

A subset of infants may indeed be prevented from successful breastfeeding unless they undergo frenotomy; however, most infants with tongue-tie can breastfeed successfully with appropriate support.

5. **Infantile dyschezia**

Many straining and crying babies who are otherwise well are unnecessarily submitted to an often-escalating regime of milk changes and laxatives despite eventually passing a soft stool. This problem is actually caused by a lack of coordination between sphincter relaxation and abdominal muscle contraction when trying to open the bowels. It almost always resolves by 6 months of age. Ensure that the baby is thriving and does not have any other abdominal symptoms such as abdominal distension, blood in the stool or bilious vomiting.

6. **KISS syndrome**

'Kinematic imbalances due to suboccipital strain', or KISS syndrome, has not yet spilt over from Germany to the mainstream here but has already managed to feature prominently on Mumsnet (www.mumsnet.com). It is blamed for a variety of ills commonly affecting young infants, from head asymmetry, through feeding problems, to excessive screaming. There is no science in this, so it is probably a non-diagnosis. If your opinion is sought and the child does have a torticollis, refer to a paediatric physiotherapist.

Easily Confused

1. Reactive lymphadenitis and lymphoma

Reactive lymphadenitis	Lymphoma
■ Predominantly young, preschool children	■ Peak in incidence in teenage years
■ Waxing and waning in size	■ Persistent growth
■ Smaller than 1.5 cm	■ Larger than 1.5 cm with no response to antibiotic treatment
■ Affecting mainly neck chains, often with an upper respiratory tract infection	■ Unusual location, especially supraclavicular nodes
■ Well between episodes of febrile illnesses	■ Weight loss, night sweats, pruritus, unexplained fevers

2. Positional plagiocephaly and premature synostosis of the cranial sutures

Positional plagiocephaly	Premature synostosis of the cranial sutures
■ Develops after birth	■ Often present at birth
■ Typical parallelogram appearance of skull with ipsilateral flattening of the occiput and bossing of frontal skull when viewed from top	■ Skull growth in direction of the fused suture
■ Ear displaced away from flattening	■ Ear displaced towards flattening
■ May be associated with developmental dysplasia of the hips, visual field defects, neuromuscular disease or sternocleidomastoid muscle shortening	■ Children may look syndromic (in about 30% of cases of premature synostosis, e.g. Crouzon syndrome)

3. Transient synovitis and septic arthritis

Transient synovitis	Septic arthritis
■ Well child	■ In the early stages may appear cranky, off feeds with low-grade fever
■ Sudden onset, typically refusing to weight-bear after waking in the morning	■ Gradual onset and progression of symptoms
■ Usually one hip joint	■ Any joint can be affected
■ Spontaneous recovery within 2 to 3 days	■ Ongoing symptoms unless treated

4. Daydreaming and absence seizures

Daydreaming	Absence seizures
■ Any age	■ Usually school age
■ Occasional episodes	■ Numerous episodes each day
■ Long duration (minutes)	■ Shorter duration (usually seconds)
■ Can be stopped (usually physically touching the child will be required)	■ Does not respond to stimuli
■ Situational: child bored	■ Can be triggered by hyperventilation

5. Paroxysmal non-epileptic events and epileptic seizures

Paroxysmal non-epileptic events	Epileptic seizures
■ Long duration (more than 5 to 10 minutes)	■ Shorter duration of convulsive phase
■ Fluctuation in motor activity and thrashing movements, tremor-like movements of limbs	■ Tonic/clonic
■ Side-to-side movement of head or body	■ Unilateral deviation, often during tonic phase
■ Eye closure during the attack and resistance to passive eye opening	■ Eyes mostly open during seizure

6. Sacral dimples and spinal dysraphism

Sacral dimples	Spinal dysraphism
■ Usually located within the natal cleft (less than 25 mm away from the anus)	■ Above upper natal cleft
■ Skin dimple (even if deep and bottom not visible), no discharge	■ Tufts of hair, pigmented macules, haemangiomata, discharge
■ Normal head circumference	■ May have hydrocephalus
■ No imaging required	■ Needs MRI for full evaluation
■ Possible complications: (Pilonidal) sinus infection, difficulties with daily hygiene	■ Possible complications: Neurological impairment (decreased reflexes), tethered cord, meningitis

Prescribing Points

1. Children are not small adults

Underlying pathophysiological mechanisms and pharmacokinetics vary greatly, not only compared to adults (effects and doses are often merely extrapolated from adult studies) but also within the paediatric age group. Prescribing is not made easier by the fact that many medications given to children are unlicensed. So, as a general rule, prescribing for children should be restrictive. First, do no harm!

2. Medications for gastro-oesophageal reflux

It is important not to reflexively react to parental anxiety by medicating the baby. First, consider whether the baby is being overfed and consider thickening feeds.

Next, consider antacid treatment for a maximum of 4 weeks, then try without. There is very little evidence for the efficacy of reflux treatments, and concerns are evolving regarding the potential harm of so-called prokinetics.

3. **Iron**

   A child that has started iron therapy should receive a course of at least 3 months to replenish iron stores. Even then, a prophylactic dose for another couple of months may be needed. Every child with iron deficiency needs serology screening for coeliac disease. If the blood film remains microcytic and hypochromic (red cell indices usually recover within a few weeks of treatment), think alpha thalassaemia trait or poor compliance.

4. **Antipyretics**

   This term is a misnomer. Drugs such as paracetamol and ibuprofen do on average reduce a raised body temperature by no more than 1.5°C, but the only reason to give analgesia (my preferred term) to ill children is to address their discomfort. By advising to give regular medication for fever to 'control' a temperature and prevent complications such as febrile seizures, one is setting parents up to fail and exposing the child to the toxicity of recurrent inappropriate medication.

PALLIATIVE CARE

Dylan Harris

Ten Pearls of Wisdom

1. **A hand-held fan will have the same benefit as oxygen for most patients with breathlessness in advanced disease**

   Breathlessness is a common symptom in advanced malignant and non-malignant diseases (prevalence 40%–80%). Most of these patients will not be hypoxic (i.e. oxygen saturations >90%), but may still report a subjective benefit from oxygen. Randomised placebo-controlled trials have not found a difference between oxygen or air through a mask in this context. Non-hypoxic patients will therefore generally find a hand-held fan as effective. This is thought to be from stimulation of the trigeminal nerve from the flow of air across the face and can avoid unnecessary dependence on oxygen.

2. **Opioid patches are not recommended first line for pain but do have a role**

   Opioid patches are not recommended first line but can be helpful for example, in severe dysphagia where there is difficulty with oral medication (e.g. head and neck cancer; advanced neurological disease), malabsorption (e.g. after extensive bowel surgery), poor tablet compliance (e.g. dementia) or risk of oral opioid misuse/diversion.

   See Table 24.1 or online (e.g. www.book.pallcare.info) for opioid conversion calculation.

3. **Choice of drug for neuropathic pain can be guided by adjuvant benefits**

   Gabapentin/pregabalin, amitriptyline/nortriptyline and duloxetine are recommended first-line options for neuropathic pain. Their efficacy is similar. Concurrent symptoms can direct towards one or other, for example, neuropathic pain with low mood and poor sleep: amitriptyline; in contrast, neuropathic pain and significant anxiety: gabapentin.

   If there is no improvement in pain with one drug in the group, then there is no rationale for trying the other option within the same group (e.g. pregabalin after gabapentin); try a different mechanism of action (e.g. gabapentin then

DOI: 10.1201/9781003304586-24

Table 24.1 Equivalent potency of transdermal opioids

Transdermal opioid	Patch strength: Equivalent total oral morphine daily dose
Buprenorphine[a]	5 µg/hour = 12 mg
	10 µg/hour = 24 mg
	20 µg/hour = 48 mg
	35 µg/hour = 84 mg
	52.5 µg/hour = 126 mg
	70 µg/hour = 168 mg
Fentanyl[a]	12 µg/hour = 43 mg
	25 µg/hour = 90 mg
	37 µg/hour = 133 mg
	50 µg/hour = 180 mg
	62 µg/hour = 223 mg
	75 µg/hour = 270 mg
	87 µg/hour = 313 mg
	100 µg/hour = 360 mg

[a] Patches can be combined to give doses between the fixed strength, for example using the fentanyl 25 µg and fentanyl 12 µg patches simultaneously (i.e. 37 µg total).

amitriptyline). Where there is some benefit from either, but titration is limited by side effects, try combining both at tolerated doses given their different methods of action (e.g. amitriptyline with gabapentin).

4. Steroids have a number of useful potential indications in palliative care

Dexamethasone is generally used because it has a lower tablet burden than equivalent doses of prednisolone.

Common uses/daily starting doses:

a. *2–4 mg*: Appetite/fatigue, nausea/vomiting
b. *4–8 mg*: Pain (by reducing peri-tumour oedema/inflammation)
c. *8–16 mg*: Malignant spinal cord compression; lymphangitis carcinomatosis; malignant bowel obstruction, cerebral oedema, superior vena cava obstruction

Generally, use should be short term, with the dose reduced by 2 mg every 5 to 7 days (to prevent longer-term side effects). Dexamethasone can be given in a syringe driver or daily subcutaneous injection (as it has a long duration of action). The latter is preferred, as dexamethasone is not compatible with other drugs in a syringe driver.

5. Driving is not an absolute barrier to starting strong opioids

UK 'drug driving' regulations specifically include driving while taking drugs such as morphine (prescribed or not). The law does allow a 'medical defence' when the drug is prescribed and taken in accordance with instructions; however, it is legally the driver's responsibility to decide whether they consider their driving is impaired on any given occasion. There are a number of patient information leaflets which give patients practical guidance, for example, not driving for 5 days after starting a long-acting opioid (or dose change), or 4 to 6 hours after a short-acting one (e.g. https://tinyurl.com/opioiddriving).

There is no specific legal restriction to a patient with a syringe driver driving, as long as it is not felt to be impairing driving ability.

6. Initiate anti-secretory agents for 'death rattle' sooner rather than later

'Death rattle' occurs in about 50% of patients at the end of life. Drugs such as hyoscine hydrobromide and glycopyrronium have similar overall efficacy (50%–66% response). Physiologically, they primarily reduce development of further secretions (rather than dissipate existing secretions), and so should be introduced sooner rather than later.

Usually, the patient is deeply unconscious at this point. It is worth explaining to the family that while the noise of the secretions is very distressing, the patient is unlikely to be aware of the problem, that is, it does not cause suffocation, choking or distress (unless the patient is clearly agitated by the secretions).

7. When asked about prognosis, talk in terms of hours to days, days to weeks or weeks to months

Answering questions about prognosis is difficult. Responses too vague – such as 'it's impossible to put a timescale on it' – do not give the patient an indication of where they are in their disease trajectory. Whereas a response may be so specific – 'the average survival from X is 2 months' – that patients firmly anticipate that exact date in the calendar. Perhaps the best balance is to respond along the lines of 'when we see that someone is notably deteriorating from week to week, then we estimate their outlook to be weeks, and when that deterioration is noticeable from day to day we are usually talking in terms of days'.

8. Remember the four A's for anticipatory prescribing

Around two-thirds of the hours in the week are 'out of hours', when a patient's GP and pharmacist are less likely to be open. Proactive prescribing of end-of-life medication 'just in case' can save significant delays in receiving medication out of hours and, in some cases, hospital admission.

This should include the four A's: analgesic (e.g. subcutaneous morphine), anti-emetic (e.g. subcutaneous cyclizine), anxiolytic (e.g. subcutaneous midazolam), anti-secretory (e.g. subcutaneous hyoscine hydrobromide).

9. **Try to identify non-cancer patients appropriate for the GP palliative care register**

   It can be difficult to identify which patients with a non-cancer life-limiting progressive illness are most appropriate to include on a GP palliative care register. For example, stage III–IV heart failure has a poorer 1-year survival than many common cancers. Several palliative care prognostic tools have *disease-specific* triggers which will help (e.g. www.tinyurl.com/GSFtool) in combination with the 'surprise question', i.e. 'would you be surprised if this patient were to die in the next 6–12 months?'

10. **Constipation is common but avoid concurrent use of several laxatives**

    Constipation is common because of multiple factors (drugs, e.g. opioids; reduced fluid intake; reduced mobility). There is no significant difference in efficacy between laxatives. A combination of a softener (e.g. magnesium hydroxide) and a stimulant (e.g. senna) is commonly used. Prescribe one or a combination of up to two to be taken regularly in sufficient quantities. The use of several laxatives concurrently adds significantly to the medication burden and makes it very difficult to establish which works 'best' for that particular patient. Macrogol laxatives require dilution in water, and the volume to be taken for an adequate daily dose can be too much for very frail patients. Patients with dementia may comply best with lactulose, presumably because of the more palatable sweet taste.

Obscure or Overlooked Diagnoses

1. **Symptom control of pruritus**

   Pruritus is a less common symptom but has a major impact on quality of life. Often, an antihistamine is given and this may be an appropriate first option; however, frequently histamine is not the primary chemical mediator of pruritus in palliative care. Other options to consider include sertraline or rifampicin for cholestasis (e.g. obstructive jaundice from a pancreatic tumour), doxepin or gabapentin for uraemia (e.g. end-stage renal failure), ondansetron for opioid-induced pruritus when an anti-histamine has not worked, and sertraline for paraneoplastic pruritus. Note that these are non-licensed indications (as with a lot of prescribing for symptom control in palliative care; see Prescribing point 4), and so are often initiated in collaboration with the local palliative care team.

2. **Malignant spinal cord compression (MSCC)**

   One in ten patients with spinal metastases will develop MSCC. Early diagnosis has a direct consequence on outcome: function will be retained in 70% of those ambulant at the point of starting treatment (radiotherapy/spinal surgery), but only in 5% of those who have already become paraplegic.

Back pain (new/escalating pain) is a red flag and vague sensory symptoms are often the initial presentation; diagnosis should not be delayed until the classic features of a sensory level and paraplegia develop. Light-touch sensation may be normal initially and pinprick sensation should always be checked. When MSCC is suspected clinically, dexamethasone should be started immediately and admission for urgent MRI arranged, unless the patient is already very frail, bedbound and has a short prognosis.

3. **Superior vena cava obstruction (SVCO)**

SVCO can have quite an insidious presentation and can easily be overlooked, particularly if the patient is already breathless – for example, from lung cancer or known lung metastases. External compression usually occurs in the region of the right main bronchus, and checking whether there is a known tumour mass or malignant lymph nodes in that area can help if uncertain. Patients may not notice collateral venous dilation on the chest wall, so it is worth looking for. Swelling of the face, neck and arms but not the legs is also a useful indicator. Intraluminal stents or oncological treatment of the underlying cause (e.g. radiotherapy) is the main treatment, as well as dexamethasone. For very frail patients not fit for further investigation, dexamethasone could be trialled at home on the basis of clinical suspicion.

4. **Brain metastases as an intracranial cause for persisting nausea**

Brain metastases can present as persistent unexplained nausea only. While the usual presentation of brain metastases would have other associated features, it is always worth bearing this in mind in a patient with known malignancy and nausea of unclear cause – actively enquire about other relevant symptoms such as headaches or visual disturbances.

Easily Confused

1. Opioid toxicity and serotonin syndrome

Opioid toxicity	Serotonin syndrome
■ Confusion, agitation, hallucinations	■ Confusion, agitation, hallucinations
■ Small or pinpoint pupils	■ Dilated pupils
■ Myoclonic jerks	■ Tremor, akathisia, may have myoclonus
■ Respiratory depression (may not be present if mild)	■ May have autonomic features, e.g. tachycardia, change in temperature/blood pressure
■ Recent deterioration in renal function or increase in opioid use	■ On a combination of implicated drugs, e.g. SSRIs, tramadol, fentanyl, metoclopramide

2. Malignant spinal cord compression and steroid myopathy

Malignant spinal cord compression	Steroid myopathy
■ Patient presenting with 'weakness' in arms and/or legs ■ Power loss but with associated sensory symptoms/ signs (pinprick may be lost before light-touch sensation) ■ Improvement with dexamethasone rather than associated with it	■ Patient presenting with 'weakness' in arms and/or legs ■ Proximal muscle power loss only, with no sensory signs ■ More likely if history of dexamethasone >4 mg daily (or prednisolone >40 mg) for more than 2 months

Prescribing Points

1. Anti-emetics
Choice of first option anti-emetic should be guided by identifying the likely cause of the nausea and selecting the anti-emetic most likely to work on the receptors which have been triggered (Table 24.2).

2. Opioid conversions
In some circumstances, it may be advisable to switch between strong opioids ('opioid rotation') – for example, in dose-limiting neurocognitive side effects

Table 24.2 Anti-emetics for nausea and vomiting in palliative care

Cause of nausea/vomiting	Preferable first-line anti-emetic options
■ Drug, toxin, metabolic cause, e.g. opioid-related nausea, hypercalcaemia	■ Haloperidol OR ■ Metoclopramide OR ■ Domperidone
■ Malignant bowel obstruction	■ If complete obstruction: hyoscine butylbromide OR cyclizine ± octreotide ■ If subacute/partial obstruction: metoclopramide
■ Chemotherapy, radiotherapy	■ Ondansetron OR ■ Granisetron
■ Raised intracranial pressure/ intracerebral cause, e.g. brain metastases	■ Cyclizine ± dexamethasone
■ Delayed gastric emptying	■ Metoclopramide OR ■ Domperidone

■ Multiple causes and where first-line option ineffective	■ *Options:*
	  ■ Try another emetic with different mechanism of action (e.g. metoclopramide instead of cyclizine)
	  ■ Some anti-emetics can be used in combination (e.g. cyclizine and haloperidol, but not metoclopramide and cyclizine)
	  ■ Use a second-line broad-spectrum anti-emetic, e.g. levomepromazine

Table 24.3 Opioid conversions

Convert from	To	By	Example: From	Approximate equivalence to
Codeine (oral)	Morphine (oral)	Divide dose by 10	Co-codamol 30/500 8/day (240 mg codeine)	24 mg oral morphine daily
Tramadol (oral)	Morphine (oral)	Divide dose by 10	Tramadol 100 mg four times daily	40 mg oral morphine daily
Morphine (oral)	Oxycodone (oral)	Divide by 2 or 1.5	Morphine sulphate tablets 40 mg twice daily (i.e. 80 mg total)	Oxycontin 20 mg twice daily (i.e. 40 mg total)
Morphine (oral)	Diamorphine (subcutaneous)	Divide by 3	Morphine sulphate tablets 15 mg twice daily (i.e. 30 mg total)	Diamorphine 10 mg/24 hours
Morphine (oral)	Morphine (subcutaneous)	Divide by 2	Morphine sulphate tablets 60 mg twice daily	Morphine 60 mg over 24 hours subcutaneously
Oxycodone (oral)	Oxycodone (subcutaneous)	Divide by 2 or 1.5	Oxycodone modified release 20 mg twice daily (i.e. 40 mg total)	Oxycodone 20 mg subcutaneously/24 hours

such as excessive somnolence, hallucinations and confusion. Conversion ratios between common opioids are shown in Table 24.3. The Palliative Adult Network Guidelines has an online opioid dose converter: www.book.pallcare.info.

3. **De-prescribing is as important as prescribing in palliative care**
   As well as adding medication for symptom control, reviewing and rationalising existing medication is essential. For example, there is no deleterious effect from stopping statins in patients with an estimated prognosis of 12 months or less.

4. **Use of drugs beyond their license ('off-label') in palliative care**
   Up to a quarter of prescriptions in palliative care are 'off-label', for example amitriptyline for neuropathic pain and haloperidol for nausea. It is important to note that the marketing authorisation for drugs largely regulates the marketing activities of pharmaceutical companies rather than restricts the prescribing practice per se, that is, use of 'established drugs for proven but unauthorised indications'. The British Pain Society and the Association for Palliative Medicine of Great Britain and Ireland have produced a useful consensus statement to support this and give further details: http://tinyurl.com/pallcareofflabel.

PSYCHIATRY

David S. Baldwin

Ten Pearls of Wisdom

1. **Be vigilant for the appearance of hypomanic or manic episodes in patients with recurrent depression**

   The 'switch' rate to bipolar disorder in patients with recurrent depression is about 1% per year of illness (i.e. a 10% chance of experiencing a first hypomanic or manic episode over 10 years). Most patients in a seemingly unipolar depressive episode do not subsequently develop bipolar illness, but some do and it is hard to distinguish between unipolar and bipolar depressive episodes. Longer sleep and increased appetite are more frequent in bipolar than unipolar depressive episodes but other features are better pointers to 'bipolarity', including early onset of illness, frequently recurring episodes, psychotic features and 'activation' while taking antidepressants. The self-description of 'being a bit bipolar' bears little relation to the incapacitating episodes of severely disturbed mood experienced by patients with bipolar disorder.

2. **Psychotic depression is more common than you might think**

   About 10% of depressive episodes are accompanied by 'mood-congruent' psychotic features. These are principally guilty, nihilistic or persecutory delusions (e.g. beliefs about deserving to be punished, of being destitute and of being hounded for supposed misdemeanours), and second-person auditory hallucinations (e.g. 'you are a worthless idiot' and 'kill yourself'). Health professionals often feel uncomfortable asking specific questions about possible psychotic features for fear of causing offence. But this can lead to serious misjudgements about illness severity, risking inappropriate treatment decisions and suicide. Become comfortable and practised in asking specific questions about psychotic features in depressed patients.

3. **The risk of suicide is greatly increased in patients with preoccupying suicidal thoughts persisting beyond the immediate aftermath of an admission for self-harm**

   Only a small proportion of those who have recently harmed themselves will take their life in the subsequent year. Yet somehow, the most suicidal patients

DOI: 10.1201/9781003304586-25

often manage to avoid psychiatric assessment before returning home after a brief hospital stay, and some of these will present to the GP. Be aware that suicide risk is increased about 100 times in patients with preoccupying suicidal thoughts continuing after a self-harm admission. But the prediction of suicide is an inexact science: the only useful predictive factors are a history of self-harm and the presence of suicidal thoughts, although most at high risk do not die by suicide, whereas some considered at low risk will.

4. Panic attacks do not equate to panic disorder, and some 'panic patients' stop experiencing panic

About 1 in 10 people experience a single panic attack, and approximately 1 in 20 will have two or more, usually at difficult times and in feared situations. Panic attacks can occur with depression and other anxiety disorders, but panic disorder is characterised by the presence of at least some attacks coming 'out of the blue'. Most patients with panic disorder have frequent episodes, but the most severely affected can become so markedly agoraphobic and housebound that panic attacks no longer occur. When judging illness severity, consider panic attack frequency, degree of anticipatory anxiety, levels of agoraphobic avoidance and symptom-related impairment, and co-existing depression.

5. Do not expect patients with schizophrenia to contact you when they are relapsing

None of us can see ourselves as others do; to some degree, we all lack insight. The ability to relabel unusual symptoms as indicators of illness is not shared universally, but patients with schizophrenia are particularly likely to choose the wrong course of action when becoming unwell. Avoidance of doctors may seem wise when previous encounters have led to hospital admissions and unwanted medications. When a patient does not attend an appointment, do not think this implies all is well; instead, try to contact the patient or their allocated community mental health practitioner.

6. Most traumatic experiences do not lead to post-traumatic stress disorder (PTSD)

To be exposed does not equate to being traumatised. About half the population will experience or witness a life-threatening event; most exposed individuals do not develop persistent or later-onset emotional symptoms, and only a minority of those who do will develop post-traumatic psychological syndromes. Trauma is more commonly followed by depression than PTSD. Encourage recently exposed patients who seem in good shape to resume routine everyday activities as soon as possible; do not attempt a 'debrief' and do not medicalise the experience. But trauma-exposed individuals with 're-experiencing' symptoms (flashbacks and nightmares) and hyperarousal, and those with depressive symptoms need careful assessment.

7. 'Hearing voices' does not necessarily indicate psychosis

Many patients who describe hearing 'voices' do not have a psychotic illness. 'True' auditory hallucinations are heard in object space (i.e. outside the body), whereas many patients hear voices 'inside their head' (i.e. in subject space, sometimes called 'pseudohallucinations'). Object space hallucinations can be a feature of acute confusional states, schizophrenia, mania and depression; whereas subject space pseudohallucinations are common in patients with personality disorders, especially those with a history of prolonged abuse during childhood. Both are distressing, but pseudohallucinations do not respond well to antipsychotic drug treatment.

8. Cognitive behaviour therapy (CBT) is not a panacea for human suffering

Many patients with anxiety or depression will derive some benefit from CBT when undertaken in sufficient sessions with trained and supervised practitioners following a structured treatment manual. Some psychotic patients become less distressed by delusions and hallucinations when undertaking CBT given in a similar manner. But too much of what is delivered as 'CBT' is unstructured and unsupervised. CBT does not help all psychiatric patients (hence the development of 'third-wave' psychological interventions, such as those based on mindfulness), and some patients report persistent negative effects of psychological treatment. Recognise that much woe and misery is not amenable to either psychological or pharmacological intervention.

9. Ask specifically about alcohol consumption in patients with depressive symptoms

The presence of an unrecognised alcohol use disorder is one of the major causes of 'treatment-resistant' depression. When compared to depressed patients without alcohol problems, depressed patients with comorbid alcoholism take twice as long to recover, have twice the risk of recurrence and are twice as likely to commit suicide. Patients often minimise their consumption, so take time to explore carefully and in detail alcohol consumption in patients with persistent depression.

10. We are all patients or potential patients

Depressive and anxiety symptoms are distributed continuously in primary care patients – most patients have only a few anxiety or depressive symptoms, but there is no clear distinction between those who 'have' depression or anxiety and those who do not. Symptoms will worsen at difficult times, then reduce as problems resolve. Doctors are patients too. If you are troubled and performing less well than usual, discuss your worries with a friend or colleague. We are mostly resilient and robust, but not superhuman: we should expect to be unsettled by unwanted change and upset by untoward events. Humility and frailty are valuable personal commodities.

Obscure or Overlooked Diagnoses

1. **Obsessive-compulsive disorder (OCD)**

   Most people describing themselves as 'a bit OCD' are merely fastidious and precise; patients with OCD typically suffer from a long-term, distressing and disabling condition. Although common, it is often overlooked, partly because patients experience shame and fear ridicule, but also because OCD is often comorbid with depression, and only the depressive symptoms are volunteered or recognised. To judge OCD severity, assess the degree of distress and associated disability of ruminations and doubts, and physical and mental rituals.

2. **Generalised anxiety disorder (GAD)**

   GAD is the most common anxiety disorder in people over 65 years old. Because patients often present with co-existing depression, and because worries about illness and the future are expected at retirement age, it is often overlooked. Depressed patients with unrecognised comorbid GAD have more severe symptoms, greater impairment, a more prolonged and recurring course of illness, and a higher risk of attempted suicide. Distinguishing between GAD and persistent unipolar depression can be difficult but is worthwhile as the two conditions are treated differently.

3. **Social anxiety disorder (social phobia)**

   'Shyness' is to social phobia what low mood is to depression; a key symptom, but only one part of a broad syndrome. The characteristically early onset (mid-teenage years) of fear and avoidance of social and performance situations is distressing and debilitating. Socially anxious patients tend to avoid authority figures such as doctors, so many do not present to their GP. Some will attend, though, often with depressive symptoms – in which case, remember to consider social anxiety.

4. **Morbid jealousy**

   Transient jealous feelings are not uncommon in loving relationships but can become fixed, preoccupying and disruptive. Morbid jealousy can be a feature of an underlying illness such as depression or alcohol dependence, though may occur in isolation. Most patients with obsessive ruminations or delusional convictions about a partner's supposed infidelity will endure a silent but wretched torment; however, escalating and ill-founded accusations of secretive sexual misdemeanours should raise significant concern. The abject and demoralised patient may kill himself, but a desperate, vengeful individual may try to kill their spouse or partner.

5. **Delusional misidentification syndromes**

   This is a varied and perplexing group, characterised by the delusional belief that the identity of a person, object or place has somehow changed. This delusion is often just one feature of an underlying illness such as psychotic depression or schizophrenia. Certain misidentification delusions are more common and known eponymously, for example Capgras delusion relates to the replacement of a close relative or spouse by a physically identical impostor. All are distressing and usually frightening, and there is an increased risk of violence.

6. **Folie à deux (shared psychosis)**

This is a shared and often long-standing condition in which a delusional belief (and sometimes a hallucination) is 'transmitted' from one person to another. It most commonly occurs in physically or socially isolated couples; one of whom is domineering (the 'inducer'), the other (the 'acceptor') more passive. Admission and treatment of the acceptor are usually only temporarily successful, as relapses occur after returning home if the inducer remains untreated. But the acceptor will usually steadily improve without the need for treatment if the inducer is separated geographically and treated successfully.

Easily Confused

1. Social anxiety disorder, and agoraphobia and panic disorder

	Social anxiety disorder	*Agoraphobia and panic disorder*
Characteristic fear	Of humiliation and embarrassment	Of being overwhelmed by anxiety where help is not available
Avoidance	■ Of social events and authority figures; abhorrence of scrutiny	■ Of situations in which panic attacks have occurred
Panic attacks	■ Typically restricted to social and performance situations	■ Typically occur when outside home or when left alone at home
Facial symptoms	■ Blushing and stuttering	■ Blanching
Supermarket checkout	■ Anxiety worsens as nears front of queue; the worst is yet to come	■ Anxiety lessens towards front of queue; it will soon all be over

2. Depressive episode and generalised anxiety disorder

	Depressive episode	*Generalised anxiety disorder*
Prevailing emotion	■ Self-loathing and remorse	■ Intolerance of uncertainty
Cognitive symptoms	■ Self-reproach and regret over past actions and choices	■ Apprehensive worries about what might occur in the future
Variation in low mood	■ Typically most profound early in the morning but brightening a little over the day	■ Some dejection when worst fears appear confirmed, brightening when again proved incorrect
Sleep disturbance	■ Middle and late insomnia	■ Initial insomnia
Suicidal thoughts	■ Common; death is welcome	■ Uncommon; death is feared

3. Psychotic depression and schizophrenia with depression

	Psychotic depression	Schizophrenia with depression
Psychotic features	■ Typically mood-congruent	■ Often both mood-congruent and mood-incongruent
Observed slowness	■ Psychomotor retardation (as if mentally and physically wading through treacle)	■ Poverty of movement (loss of desire and appreciation of need to undertake activities)
Delusional beliefs	■ Guilty, nihilistic (and persecutory)	■ All types may occur
Auditory hallucinations	■ Second person, brief – e.g. 'you worthless fool'	■ Third person, prolonged – e.g. 'he eats his soup like a girl but dresses like a chameleon'
Suicidal acts	■ Typically premeditated and carefully planned	■ Often impulsive and reckless

Prescribing Points

1. **Metabolic syndrome and psychotropic drugs**
   'Metabolic syndrome' can arise during antipsychotic and antidepressant drug treatment. It is also seen in untreated patients with schizophrenia and bipolar disorder. NICE guidance recommends regular physical health monitoring in patients with severe mental illness. Screen annually for diabetes and other cardiovascular risk factors, and actively manage weight gain.
2. **Sexual dysfunctions associated with antidepressants**
   Sexual adverse effects of SSRI and SNRIs are common (approximately 40% of male and female patients) and may affect treatment adherence. The most common effects are delayed ejaculation, anorgasmia in women and reduced sexual desire. Some patients improve with dose reduction or switching to another antidepressant (such as agomelatine or bupropion, both best done in secondary care).
3. **Sweating with the SNRI venlafaxine**
   Excess perspiration with venlafaxine can be very bothersome and may make some patients want to stop treatment. It probably arises from an unbalanced inhibition of the reuptake of serotonin and noradrenaline. For duloxetine (another SNRI) this is more balanced, and some patients who sweat profusely with venlafaxine will become cool and serene if switched to duloxetine.
4. **Starting and monitoring long-term lithium treatment**
   Decisions to start lithium are best made in secondary care. Monitor lithium levels and renal and thyroid function every 3 to 6 months, and wherever possible avoid combining lithium with diuretics, NSAIDs or ACE inhibitors.

Warn against suddenly stopping treatment, because of 'rebound' mania. Early symptoms of toxicity include worsening tremor, vomiting and diarrhoea; later signs include disorientation, dysarthria and convulsions. In suspected toxicity, withhold the next dose and perform urgent lithium level and renal function; refer to A&E if features are severe.

5. **Lamotrigine is useful in many patients with bipolar disorder**
   Although the necessarily incremental dosage escalation can be a challenge, daily doses between 150 and 400 mg can be effective in reducing the likelihood of further episodes of illness, particularly depressive episodes. Regular estimation of blood levels is not required, and weight gain and drowsiness during treatment are uncommon. But patients need to be warned about the risk of nasty skin eruptions and must stop treatment should any rashes occur. Best started in secondary care.

6. **Risk of non-prescribed use with gabapentin or pregabalin**
   Within the UK, gabapentin is not licensed for treating patients with psychiatric disorders, but pregabalin can be effective in short-term treatment and relapse prevention in generalised anxiety disorder (licensed indication) and social anxiety disorder (unlicensed). However, gabapentin and pregabalin abuse is reported, particularly in patients with substance use disorders, and the drug has street value. Avoid gabapentin and pregabalin in patients with a history of drug abuse and beware of early requests for repeat prescriptions.

7. **Withdrawal of benzodiazepines**
   Although it is tempting to use antidepressants or beta-blockers to 'manage' anxiety while benzodiazepines are withdrawn, the evidence for doing so is limited. The best approach is gradual dosage reduction, at a rate felt comfortable by the patient, coupled with simple psychological techniques based on goal-setting, encouragement and support.

8. **Neuroleptic malignant syndrome**
   A rare but sometimes fatal neuropsychiatric condition characterised by a decreased consciousness level, muscular rigidity, hyperthermia and labile blood pressure. It can occur at any time during treatment, evolves rapidly (over days) and often persists (10–14 days) if left untreated. Rhabdomyolysis can lead to renal failure and death. Patients should be admitted. Look for other features of the condition when patients on antipsychotics present with fever.

9. **Serotonin syndrome**
   This rare but potentially fatal condition is characterised by confusion, pyrexia, sweating, myoclonic jerks, hyper-reflexia and gastrointestinal disturbance, typically emerging over a few hours. It is most frequently described when an SSRI or SNRI has been co-prescribed with other drugs that enhance serotonin bioavailability (such as monoamine oxidase inhibitors or tramadol). Symptoms usually resolve promptly after drug withdrawal, but severe forms need hospital referral. Avoid combining SSRIs or SNRIs with tramadol.

10. **Symptoms experienced while reducing and after stopping antidepressants**
    Stopping an antidepressant abruptly can be followed by disturbed sleep,
    increased nervousness and gastrointestinal symptoms (common), and sensory
    and motor complaints (less common). Symptoms typically emerge within 2
    days, reach peak intensity after around 5 days and then resolve gradually, but
    some patients report severe and distressing symptoms which persist for many
    months. Discontinuation symptoms may be more severe with paroxetine and
    venlafaxine, but are relatively mild with fluoxetine. When planning to withdraw
    antidepressants, tapering the dose down is generally advised, though the evidence
    for this is mixed.

RENAL MEDICINE

Aroon Lal and Tom Hughes

Ten Pearls of Wisdom

1. Interpret eGFR and creatinine carefully

The estimated glomerular filtration rate (eGFR) is calculated from the plasma
creatinine, age and sex of the patient using a complex mathematical formula. It
is no longer adjusted for ethnicity. A mild to moderate elevation of creatinine
(and reduction in eGFR) may be due to an increased release from muscles
(large muscle bulk, vigorous exercise or even a large protein meal). If the result
is unexpected, repeat a fasting measurement 2 weeks later (more urgently if
the dysfunction is marked, the patient is unwell, or the urine tests positive for
blood and/or protein) before considering a renal referral. Remember the eGFR
calculation is not validated in paediatric or pregnant patients, patients with
extremes of size or muscle mass, limb amputations, or patients with AKI. Finally,
the accuracy of laboratory creatinine assays is $\pm 5\%$, so bear this in mind when
interpreting results.

2. Unprovoked hypokalaemia is an indicator of possible secondary hypertension

Patients with a new diagnosis of hypertension should have a baseline biochemistry
and urinalysis to exclude renal disease. A low, or low normal, potassium result
should raise the possibility of an underlying cause for hypertension, particularly
if the patient is under 30 years old. Both renal artery stenosis (listen for renal or
abdominal bruits) and Conn's syndrome may be the explanation. Other rare causes
of hypertension with hypokalaemia include Cushing's syndrome (look for other
features), adrenal tumours and, in the young patient, tubular disorders such as
Liddle's syndrome. These will require specialist assessment.

3. Advise your patients to withhold ACE inhibitors/ARBs during acute illness

ACE inhibitors/angiotensin receptor blockers (ARBs) have specific effects on the
kidney, reducing efferent glomerular arteriolar resistance and lowering glomerular
filtration pressure. This forms the basis of their reno-protective, anti-proteinuric
properties, but interferes with the mechanism for maintaining glomerular

DOI: 10.1201/9781003304586-26

filtration in the event of loss of circulating volume when acute kidney injury can occur. Patients on ACE inhibitors/ARBs should omit these drugs if they develop an acute illness such as infection or gastrointestinal illness lasting more than 24 hours and should seek immediate medical advice. Diuretics, metformin and SGLT2 inhibitors should also be omitted during acute illness.

4. Proteinuria is a crucial component of CKD assessment

Dipstick proteinuria originates either from post-renal inflammatory causes such as stones, malignancy, infection, and obstruction, or from intrinsic renal causes. There are usually clinical or radiological clues for post-renal causes. If the proteinuria is of renal origin, obtaining urinary protein quantification using the urinary albumin-to-creatinine ratio (ACR) is invaluable as another marker of renal dysfunction. The majority of renal proteinuria is due to glomerular diseases such as diabetes, hypertension or glomerulonephritis. The proteinuria leads to further renal damage from inflammation and fibrosis. Management using ACE inhibitor and ARB medications reduces intraglomerular pressure and proteinuria and slows this process. SGLT2 inhibitors also achieve this, improve glycaemic control and have significant cardioprotective benefits. They are used not only for diabetes but also for CKD and heart disease.

5. Always check for a palpable bladder in patients with renal impairment

Bladder outflow obstruction is a common cause of renal dysfunction, particularly in men. So, on discovering impaired renal function, always check for urinary outflow symptoms, although these may not always be present or volunteered. Also, before requesting further investigations, examine these patients carefully for an enlarged bladder as evidence of incomplete bladder emptying – relief of the obstruction via a urinary catheter is often all that is required to improve renal function, sometimes back to normal. Such patients should be referred to urological services; they will only require a nephrology assessment if they are left with significant CKD despite relief of the obstruction.

6. Know the referral guidance for CKD

There are clear NICE guidelines on referral for renal assessment. Patients with evidence of vasculitis, acute kidney injury, nephrotic syndrome, haematuria with proteinuria (ACR >30 mg/mmol) or new CKD stage 4+ should be referred urgently. For other CKD patients, refer if they have a sustained decrease in eGFR of 25% or more within 12 months with a change in CKD category, a decrease in eGFR of 15 mL/min per year, or a 5-year risk of needing dialysis more than 5% (use the Kidney Failure Risk Equation [KFRE]). Hypertension in young patients, inherited renal conditions or isolated proteinuria (ACR >70 mg/mmol) not part of managed diabetes warrant referral. Requesting an ultrasound scan at the referral hospital (rather than alternative providers) can help to expedite the diagnosis.

7. Regardless of the cause of renal stones, the basic treatment is the same

Renal stone disease is common, affecting about 19% of men and 9% of women by the age of 70. Although exact knowledge of the chemical composition can guide treatment, the basic therapy is similar for all stone types. Patients should be advised to restrict sodium intake (advise them not to add salt to their food and to reduce their consumption of processed food and bread), and maintain a fluid intake of 2000 mL/day, including a generous drink of water before bed. Although 80% of stones contain calcium, dietary calcium restriction is ineffective. Young patients or recurrent stone formers should be referred, and the patient should be encouraged to retrieve the calculus so that it can be sent for analysis to guide more specific treatment.

8. Most renal cysts are benign and clinically insignificant

Renal cysts are a relatively common finding in patients having ultrasound scans. They are characterised radiologically using the Bosniak classification. Class I and II (thin-walled with no or only a few fine septa, of uniform attenuation and non-enhancing) require no further investigation and are rarely the cause of physical symptoms. Any other appearance of a cyst, or signs of obstruction from any cause, should prompt a urological referral. A renal opinion is required only if there are appearances of polycystic kidneys (up to 25% of patients will have no family history) or other inherited cystic disease (tuberose sclerosis, von Hippel–Lindau disease, medullary cystic disease).

9. Anaemia and CKD do not mean 'renal anaemia'

Although CKD causes a reduction in erythropoietin production and anaemia, this is not usually clinically significant until patients reach CKD stage 4 (patients with diabetes can sometimes develop anaemia in stage 3B). Patients with evidence of anaemia in earlier stages should have a full assessment, including measurement of ferritin, vitamin B_{12} and folate. Because ferritin is elevated in inflammation, transferrin saturation can be a more useful marker of iron stores, and Tsats >20 % suggests the patient is iron replete. Patients with CKD have a functional resistance to iron, so aim for ferritin levels of above 100 μg/L with oral iron supplementation. The target haemoglobin level in CKD is 100–110 g/L and initiation of erythropoiesis-stimulating agents is not indicated at levels above this.

10. Urinalysis is a simple and informative test in most patients with renal disease

Analysis of the urine can give clues to the origin of renal disease. In patients with visible haematuria, especially those with urinary symptoms, an urgent urology referral is warranted unless the haematuria resolves with successful treatment of an underlying urinary tract infection. In those with non-visible haematuria, urological causes and urinary tract infections are rarely associated with significant proteinuria (urine ACR >30 mg/mmol or 2+ on dipstick) – the presence of both haematuria and proteinuria suggests intrinsic renal disease and should prompt referral, particularly if renal impairment is present. Persistent leucocyturia with low-grade proteinuria despite antibiotic treatment may indicate tubulointerstitial disease and a renal referral should be considered, particularly in the presence of abnormal renal function. Patients with advanced CKD, in particular those on renal replacement therapy, commonly have persistent urinary abnormalities – the finding of an abnormal dip may not indicate a urinary tract infection without formal culture results, together with urinary symptoms.

Obscure and Overlooked Diagnoses

1. **Exercise-induced haematuria**
   Vigorous exercise is a recognised cause of non-visible and occasionally visible haematuria. Even if suspected, patients should have a full assessment to rule out systemic disease, including urinalysis to exclude proteinuria. The haematuria should resolve within one week if the patient refrains from exercise. If persistent or recurrent and particularly in those aged over 50 years, consider cystoscopy to exclude bladder pathology. One specific form of exercise-induced 'haematuria' is 'march haemoglobinuria'. This is thought to result from the traumatic haemolysis of red cells in the feet of long-distance runners. The urine is red-brown and tests positive for haemoglobin/red cells – but microscopy shows no visible red cells as it is not blood but haemoglobin that is being detected. If myalgia is present, blood should be sent for creatine kinase to rule out rhabdomyolysis.

2. **Orthostatic proteinuria**
   Orthostatic or postural proteinuria is the development of elevated urinary protein excretion in the upright position. It is a common cause of proteinuria in children and adolescents but is rare after the age of 30. The diagnosis is confirmed by comparing a urinary ACR taken first thing in the morning with one taken later in the day. Orthostatic proteinuria is benign and patients should be reassured.

3. **Proton pump inhibitors and tubulointerstitial nephritis**
   PPI-associated tubulointerstitial nephritis has an incidence of approximately 12/100,000 person/years of treatment. Onset is typically 2 to 4 months after commencing treatment with a gradual fall in eGFR, which may be associated with non-specific symptoms such as anorexia, weakness and myalgia. The urine may be normal, or show a trace of protein and leucocytes. Withdrawal of the

drug usually results in resolution of the renal impairment, although specialist advice should be sought.

4. **Autosomal dominant polycystic kidney disease (ADPKD)**

This affects between 1 in 400 and 1 in 1,000 births, although only about half will have the diagnosis made during their lifetime. Cysts develop in the late teens and early 20s, so ultrasound screening of family members should not be conducted until the patient is over 18. There are well-defined criteria for ultrasound diagnosis, so document the family history on the scan request. Patients may complain of flank pain from infected cysts, sometimes associated with visible haematuria. Most patients also have hypertension. All ADPKD patients should be referred for monitoring, as tolvaptan has been shown to reduce progression before the eGFR falls below 60 mL/min.

Easily Confused

1. Heart failure and nephrotic syndrome

Heart failure	Nephrotic syndrome
■ History of heart disease	■ Usually no history of heart disease
■ Gradual onset over months	■ Subacute or acute onset over days to weeks
■ Swelling confined to feet/lower legs	■ Swelling may affect hands and face, particularly first thing in the morning
■ May be precipitated by an acute cardiac event	■ May be precipitated by acute viral illness
■ Dyspnoea common	■ Dyspnoea rare
■ JVP raised	■ JVP not raised
■ Urine dip normal	■ Heavy proteinuria
■ Renal function usually normal	■ Renal function may be impaired
■ Serum albumin normal	■ Serum albumin reduced

2. Viral illness and vasculitis

Viral illness	Vasculitis
■ Acute onset	■ Insidious onset over weeks or months
■ History of contact with other affected individuals	■ No history of contact
■ Upper respiratory symptoms predominate, some myalgia and rarely arthralgia	■ Predominant symptoms are arthralgia and myalgia, anorexia and weight loss
■ Fever common	■ Usually apyrexial
■ Rash unusual, may be transient and exanthematous	■ Rash common, typically non-blanching macular, papular or purpuric, and often on the lower limbs
■ Urine dip: trace or 1+ proteinuria	■ Urine dip: haematuria and proteinuria
■ CRP mildly elevated	■ CRP significantly elevated
■ Renal function normal	■ Renal function abnormal

3. Renal calculi and primary loin pain haematuria syndrome

Renal calculi	Primary loin pain haematuria syndrome
■ Common	■ Rare (<0.1% of population)
■ Male > female	■ Female > male
■ Typically middle aged	■ Typically young adult
■ Unilateral loin pain	■ Begins unilaterally, typically bilateral
■ Visible haematuria may be present during pain	■ Visible haematuria typical during pain
■ Urine dip normal when asymptomatic	■ Non-visible haematuria usually persistent
■ Renal imaging with CT/ultrasound usually demonstrates calcification	■ Imaging normal
■ Treat with increased fluids, salt restriction and urological assessment	■ Treat with increased fluids, ACE inhibition/ARB therapy and analgesia

Prescribing Points

1. **Always check the BNF**

   Renal excretion is important for a vast number of drugs and it is impossible to commit these to memory. It is advised that everyone consult the BNF before prescribing any drug to a patient with an eGFR of below 45 mL/min.

2. **Prescribing in renal transplant patients**

   Most transplanted patients are taking calcineurin inhibitors (CNIs; specifically ciclosporin or tacrolimus) and these have important drug interactions. Diltiazem and macrolide antibiotics reduce their metabolism and may lead to toxicity, including acute renal impairment. The metabolism of statins (excluding pravastatin and fluvastatin) is reduced by CNIs and can lead to rhabdomyolysis. Simvastatin should not be used at doses higher than 10–20 mg/day and atorvastatin should be used with caution – pravastatin is preferred. Patients taking azathioprine are at risk of severe myelosuppression if given allopurinol.

3. **Treatment of UTIs in renal disease**

   a. Be cautious in prescribing trimethoprim in patients with an eGFR under 30 mL/min. Trimethoprim blocks tubular secretion of creatinine in the proximal tubule, which can cause an apparent worsening of eGFR. It also blocks potassium excretion in the distal tubule risking significant hyperkalaemia.

   b. Be cautious in prescribing nitrofurantoin to patients with an eGFR under 45 mL/min. It is relatively ineffective in CKD and systemic toxicity is increased.

4. **Analgesia in CKD**

   a. NSAIDs are relatively contraindicated in patients with an eGFR <30 mL/min (their use in patients on renin–angiotensin blocking agents is particularly risky).

   b. Most opiate metabolites undergo renal excretion. They should be used in low doses with increased dosing intervals and close monitoring. Oxycodone and fentanyl are safer alternatives.

5. **ACE inhibitors/ARBs and proteinuria**

   ACE inhibitors/ARBs are key treatments in patients with chronic kidney disease but risk worsening renal function (NICE guidance states an increase of up to 30% in creatinine is acceptable but continued deterioration should be excluded by a repeat test after a further 1–2 weeks). The evidence for the effect of these drugs is only in those with renal impairment *and* proteinuria. Exercise caution before introducing such drugs in patients with stable renal disease and *controlled* hypertension, particularly in the absence of proteinuria, for fear of doing more harm than good.

6. **Treatment of gout in CKD**

   Gout is common in patients with CKD.

   Acute attacks

   a. NSAIDs are relatively contraindicated.

   b. Colchicine doses should not exceed 500 μg bd and the duration should be limited.

   c. Glucocorticoids, either orally or in the form of a low-dose depot injection, are effective.

   Prophylaxis

   a. Prolonged administration of colchicine at doses not exceeding 500 μg daily (alternate days if eGFR <30) may help.

   b. The starting dose of allopurinol should be 100 mg daily and increments made in 50 mg steps. Doses of more than 300 mg should be avoided. The minimum dose that renders the patient free of attacks should be the aim rather than a specific urate level, as this is often unachievable.

RESPIRATORY MEDICINE

Jay Suntharalingam

Ten Pearls of Wisdom

1. **Always think twice before diagnosing COPD in a light or never smoker**

   In the developed world, the commonest cause of COPD is tobacco smoking. Damage starts in genetically susceptible individuals from their very first cigarette but, given how much reserve the lungs hold, patients tend only to become symptomatic once significant lung destruction has accumulated. This usually occurs after a 25–30 pack/year history (where 1 pack year = 20 cigarettes/day for 1 year), with patients typically presenting in their late 50s, initially with frequent bouts of 'winter bronchitis', followed by worsening exertional dyspnoea. Although patients with a lighter smoking history can develop COPD in the setting of alpha 1 antitrypsin deficiency, COPD in the absence of a significant smoking history is unusual in the majority of individuals.

2. **If an asthmatic is using >3 reliever devices per year, they likely have poorly controlled disease**

   Asthma is a common eosinophilic-driven airway disease that often affects young individuals with an atopic and/or positive family history. Airway inflammation in asthma causes airway narrowing and an increased propensity to bronchospasm, leading to wheeze, cough and breathlessness. Although patients gain short-term relief after use of a short-acting bronchodilator such as salbutamol, this only addresses the bronchospastic component in isolation and not the underlying airway inflammation. Patients who rely on their rescue inhaler more than one to two times a week require further review, focusing on inhaler technique, compliance and optimisation of their preventative medication.

3. **Oral steroids are not usually the right answer for acutely breathless patients**

   Many patients with acute breathlessness are given oral steroids, but this is often not indicated. Although oral steroids can rapidly reduce airway inflammation

DOI: 10.1201/9781003304586-27

in acute asthma exacerbations, a well-controlled asthmatic ideally should never reach the point of exacerbating. Systemic steroid courses do have a role in COPD exacerbations, but their impact is much less significant than in asthma – steroids in COPD at best shorten exacerbations by just one day. There is never an indication for steroids in acute bronchitis or pneumonia. Although steroids are occasionally used in exacerbations of pulmonary fibrosis, once infection has been excluded, this should only be instigated by a secondary care team.

4. **Always consider bronchiectasis in patients with recurrent lower respiratory tract infections**
   In bronchiectasis, patients develop dilated airways, usually following an infective insult earlier in life or as a manifestation of an underlying immunodeficiency state. Mucus pools in these dilated airways, especially at night, and becomes chronically colonised. At times, colonising organisms multiply and trigger an infective exacerbation. Bronchiectatic patients often complain of a chronic productive cough for many years, especially first thing in the morning, and frequent exacerbations, when their sputum both increases in volume and changes in colour. Patients can often outwardly look reasonably well but will typically return for multiple courses of antibiotics. A high-resolution CT (HRCT) scan can either confirm or refute the presence of bronchiectasis, whereas sputum cultures are often positive for pathogenic organisms such as *Haemophilus influenza*, *Streptococcus pneumonia* or *Moraxella catarrhalis*.

5. **If you hear inspiratory crepitations, consider idiopathic pulmonary fibrosis (IPF)**
   With advances in chest imaging and the increasing use of remote consultations, it is easy to forget the value of chest auscultation. One area in which the stethoscope remains invaluable is idiopathic pulmonary fibrosis (IPF), a common form of interstitial lung disease. The 'textbook' IPF patient is male, more than 65 years old and clubbed, with fine 'Velcro-like' inspiratory crepitations heard bilaterally. Patients eventually develop restrictive spirometry but can have normal readings early in the disease. Similarly, chest X-rays can miss early fibrotic change, whereas an HRCT of the thorax carries excellent sensitivity at any stage. It is particularly important to diagnose IPF now that antifibrotic medications such as nintedanib and pirfenidone are available that can alter its natural history.

6. **Know what to do when an echo shows evidence of pulmonary hypertension (PH)**
   Breathlessness can be due to respiratory or cardiac disease, and so all breathless patients should be screened with a serum NT-proBNP. If elevated, an echocardiogram is usually performed, which may in turn show evidence

of pulmonary hypertension (PH). More than 95% of PH is 'secondary', i.e. driven by left heart issues (i.e. 'post-capillary PH') or respiratory pathology (i.e. 'cor pulmonale') in which case treatment is targeted at the underlying cardiorespiratory condition. It is important though not to miss rare but treatable forms of 'pre-capillary' PH, such as idiopathic pulmonary arterial hypertension (IPAH; typically women in their 30s to 50s), scleroderma-associated pulmonary arterial hypertension and chronic thromboembolic pulmonary hypertension (CTEPH; see the 'Obscure or overlooked diagnoses' section for more information). If these conditions are suspected or the PH is unexplained refer.

7. If a patient has red-flag symptoms, consider a CT, even if the chest X-ray is normal

Lung cancer is often diagnosed late, such that it is now one of the highest causes of cancer-related deaths. Although smoking is a significant risk factor, up to a fifth of lung cancer cases occur in never smokers. Always consider lung cancer in any patient who presents with new breathlessness, cough, weight loss, fatigue or haemoptysis. Although a chest X-ray is adequate when the index of suspicion is low, a CT is mandated in high-risk patients, as chest X-rays can miss cancer in up to 20% of cases. CT screening is now being piloted in at-risk asymptomatic patients and is likely to become standard practice across the UK in the future.

8. Incidental pulmonary nodules often need CT surveillance

With the current widespread use of CT in medicine, it is becoming increasingly common to identify small incidental pulmonary nodules when looking for other pathology. Although many of these nodules will turn out to be benign, a small minority represent early lung cancers, offering the potential for opportunistic curative resection. In the absence of an existing malignancy, nodules measuring <5 mm are typically disregarded. All patients with nodules ≥5 mm should be referred to secondary care, as they will either need CT surveillance, potentially for up to 4 years or, in the case of larger nodules (≥8 mm), immediate investigation with PET-CT.

9. Asbestos-related pleural plaques in asymptomatic patients do not require further investigations

Asbestos was widely used in the 1950s–1960s as an insulating material in many industries, leaving a large cohort of individuals who have a history of working within an asbestos-rich environment. Asbestos exposure can cause many respiratory issues later in life, including lung cancer, mesothelioma, diffuse pleural thickening, benign pleural effusions, asbestosis and pleural plaque disease. The latter is a benign phenomenon and is often incidentally detected on chest X-rays arranged for other indications. In the absence of any red-flag symptoms (e.g. chest pain, weight loss, breathlessness or haemoptysis), patients can simply be reassured that no further investigations or onward referral is required.

10. **Don't forget to consider obstructive sleep apnoea hypopnoea syndrome (OSAHS) in patients complaining of 'tiredness'**

Obstructive sleep apnoea hypopnoea syndrome (OSAHS) describes the presence of both apnoeic spells at night, due to intermittent collapse of the upper airway, and daytime hypersomnolence. Patients report disruptive snoring with or without certain risk factors, including a large collar size, a high BMI, poor sleep hygiene, alcohol excess and a narrowed oropharynx. Individual apnoeic events are not life-threatening but, if frequent enough, can cause poor-quality sleep, leading to excessive daytime sleepiness. Investigation with sleep studies, with a view to overnight CPAP, is only indicated in those who are symptomatic, i.e. those with an Epworth Sleepiness Scale (ESS) score ≥13/24. Patients with confirmed OSAHS are required to inform the DVLA but are usually able to continue driving if established on effective treatment.

Obscure or Overlooked Diagnoses

1. **Chronic thromboembolic pulmonary hypertension (CTEPH)**

CTEPH is a treatable form of 'pre-capillary' PH that develops following an acute thromboembolic event. Clots fail to disperse and evolve into fibrotic scarring that progressively occludes the pulmonary vasculature, leading to elevated pulmonary arterial pressures. The disease can be cured with pulmonary endarterectomy surgery, while patients who have inoperable disease can improve with angioplasty and/or medication. Consider the diagnosis in patients who remain breathless months or even years after a thromboembolic event, but also be aware that about 40% of cases occur in the absence of a documented preceding event – a ventilation–perfusion (VQ) scan carries almost 100% sensitivity for identifying the disease but can give false positive results.

2. **Rheumatological disease-associated respiratory conditions**

Rheumatological conditions can be associated with a number of respiratory diseases. Many, such as rheumatoid arthritis, scleroderma and polymyositis, can directly trigger interstitial lung disease. A few, particularly systemic sclerosis and systemic lupus erythematosus (SLE), can be associated with pulmonary hypertension. In addition, drugs used to manage rheumatological conditions, such as methotrexate, can cause iatrogenic interstitial lung changes. In patients with known rheumatological disease who present with respiratory symptoms, always consider a chest X-ray and/or CT and echocardiography.

3. Hypersensitivity pneumonitis (HP)

Hypersensitivity pneumonitis (HP) is a form of interstitial lung disease that results from an allergic reaction to repeated organic dust exposure. Previously known as extrinsic allergic alveolitis (EAA), the disease is seen in certain occupations and hobbies, with avian protein exposure being one of the commonest causes. Examination can reveal inspiratory 'squawks', while CT shows characteristic features. Treatment, which can be curative, requires permanent antigen withdrawal and, in severe cases, a prolonged course of steroids.

Easily Confused

1. COPD and asthma

Both COPD and asthma are airway diseases and share several common features. It is important, however, to try to distinguish one from the other, as this will govern early use of anti-inflammatory medication (in asthma) over bronchodilator therapy (in COPD).

	COPD	**Asthma**
Age of onset <50	Rare	Common
Smoking history	Inevitable ≥25 pack/year	Possible
Family history	Rare (in absence of alpha 1 antitrypsin deficiency)	Common
Atopic history	No	Common
Cough	Productive	Dry
Nocturnal symptoms	Rare	Common
Variable breathlessness	No	Yes
Obstructive spirometry with reversibility	No	Yes
Elevated FeNO	No	Yes
Eosinophilia	No	Common

2. Inducible laryngeal obstruction (ILO) and asthma

Inducible laryngeal obstruction (ILO), previously referred to as vocal cord dysfunction (VCD) or dysfunctional breathing, describes a condition in which patients experience inappropriate laryngeal closure in response to external triggers. The condition can mimic asthma, potentially leading to unnecessary medical treatment. Once diagnosed, ILO is typically referred to a speech and language therapist for further management.

	ILO	*Asthma*
Triggers	Odours, fumes	Known allergens
Speed of onset of symptoms	Seconds	Minutes
Symptoms	Throat discomfort/voice changes	Chest tightness
Breath sounds	High-pitched grating inspiratory upper airway noise	Expiratory wheeze, heard best on chest auscultation
Response to inhalers	Poor	Good
Psychiatric comorbidities	Often present	Often absent

Prescribing Points

1. **Theophylline is no longer commonly used in asthma or COPD**
   Although theophylline has traditionally been used in both asthma and COPD, its use has fallen as other newer therapies have been introduced. Theophylline also interacts with many other medications, including antibiotics, making its use challenging. It is no longer common practice to start patients on theophylline.

2. **LAMAs have a role in asthma**
   Although long-acting muscarinic antagonist (LAMA) inhalers were initially developed for use in COPD, evidence now shows they can be effective in asthma, improving exercise tolerance and reducing exacerbation rates. They are typically used in patients who remain symptomatic despite a high-dose LABA/ICS inhaler.

3. **Biologic therapy has revolutionised asthma management for selected patients**
   Asthma patients with an eosinophilic or IgE-mediated phenotype can experience a dramatic improvement in their asthma control with the use of biologic therapies. Current guidance restricts these to patients who are steroid-dependent or who experience ≥3 exacerbations/year requiring oral steroids. Always refer patients with poorly controlled disease to secondary care so that biologic therapy can be considered.

4. **Always aim to practice good inhaler stewardship**
   The best inhaler for a patient is the one that they can use most effectively. Where patients are able to use a range of devices always aim to use a dry powdered inhaler (DPI) over a metered dose inhaler (MDI), as these are more environmentally friendly. For the same reason, try to combine inhalers wherever possible.

5. **Prophylactic azithromycin can be very effective in both COPD and bronchiectasis**

   Frequently exacerbating COPD and bronchiectasis patients can see a reduction in their exacerbations with prophylactic low-dose azithromycin. The mechanism of action is not fully understood but is thought to be due to azithromycin's anti-inflammatory, rather than antibiotic, effect. A decision to start azithromycin should initially be triggered by secondary care.

6. **Consider carbocisteine for patients with difficulty expectorating**

   Many patients with COPD, bronchiectasis and viral bronchitis intermittently experience difficulty expectorating, potentially aggravating their breathlessness through sputum plugging. Carbocisteine can provide effective symptom relief while being typically well tolerated. Some patients will benefit from remaining on carbocisteine long term, varying their dose to keep their symptoms at bay.

7. **Excessive nebulised salbutamol can precipitate lactic acidosis**

   High-dose nebulised salbutamol can trigger anaerobic metabolism, leading to profound lactic acidosis. This in turn can precipitate compensatory hyperventilation and worsen breathlessness. In acute asthma exacerbations, always use 2.5 mg nebules, rather than 5 mg nebules, and limit usage, especially if patients seem to paradoxically worsen with treatment.

RHEUMATOLOGY

Dalia Ludwig, Charlotte Wing and Jessica J. Manson

Ten Pearls of Wisdom

1. ### Inflammatory arthritis is a clinical diagnosis – do not rely on blood tests

   Patients with synovitis or inflammatory sounding joint pain should be referred to an Early Arthritis Service, even if they have normal inflammatory markers and negative autoantibodies. All blood tests can be normal in patients with rheumatoid arthritis. The pain of inflammatory arthritis is worse in the morning and with inactivity, and is associated with early morning stiffness lasting 30 minutes or more. Examination will reveal tender and/or swollen joints with synovitis, which can be difficult to detect. Look for extra-articular features of inflammatory arthritis, such as rash, nail changes, nodules, uveitis and pulmonary fibrosis.

2. ### Exclude septic arthritis when a patient presents with a single hot swollen joint

   If in any doubt about a patient presenting with a single hot swollen joint, refer urgently to exclude septic arthritis. In primary care, the usual differential is gout, but the two conditions can be difficult to distinguish (see the 'Easily confused' section). Inflammatory arthritis is a risk factor for septic arthritis, so if a patient with known inflammatory arthritis presents with a single hot swollen joint, a septic joint must still be excluded – discuss with secondary care. Similarly, if apparent cellulitis presents over a joint and there is joint pain or swelling, consider whether the joint itself could be involved. Undertreating septic arthritis could result in chronic, irreversible damage to the joint.

3. ### Have a low threshold of suspicion for sepsis in a patient on immunosuppressive therapy

   Immunosuppression from long-term steroids, disease-modifying anti-rheumatic drugs (DMARDs) and biological therapies can put patients at higher risk of infection. Bear in mind that patients on these therapies may present atypically when septic, for example, without markedly raised temperature, white cell count or C-reactive protein. If infection is a possibility, arrange appropriate

DOI: 10.1201/9781003304586-28

investigations (such as sputum/urine culture, chest X-ray) and start antibiotics promptly. If the patient appears acutely unwell, or if in doubt, discuss with the patient's rheumatologist. Immunosuppressed patients should have a yearly influenza vaccine and the pneumococcal vaccine, and have been eligible for early/ additional vaccines against COVID-19.

4. Refer urgently if you suspect possible giant cell arteritis

Giant cell arteritis (GCA) is a sight-threatening medical emergency. Most rheumatology departments will see patients with suspected GCA the same or the following day – start corticosteroids if there are any delays. Making the diagnosis conclusively involves a combination of clinical assessment, imaging (including temporal/axillary artery ultrasound and in some cases PET-CT) and laboratory tests. These initial tests are best performed within 3 days of symptom onset, as their sensitivity wanes quickly once steroids are commenced. If the diagnosis remains uncertain, a temporal artery biopsy is performed, but the abnormalities frequently resolve within 2 weeks of starting steroids. The history is fundamental in making this diagnosis, as even in the correct time frame, the tests can be normal. Giant cell arteritis is rare in patients under 60 years old. Key symptoms include headache, visual disturbance and jaw claudication. General malaise and polymyalgic symptoms may be present, and tenderness over the course of the temporal artery is suggestive. Inflammatory markers (ESR and CRP) are usually raised, but not always (see the 'Easily confused' section).

5. Reconsider the diagnosis if polymyalgia rheumatica fails to respond quickly to steroids

Polymyalgia rheumatica (PMR) is characterised by proximal limb girdle stiffness (without weakness), worse in the mornings and improving with exercise/movement – usually in those over 50. Although associated with raised inflammatory markers, there is no diagnostic test, so the diagnosis is clinical. This requires the exclusion of 'polymyalgia mimics' such as malignancy, infection, other inflammatory rheumatic diseases, and endocrine and neurological diseases. PMR characteristically responds rapidly to prednisolone 15 mg daily. Patients who fail to respond well, who require higher doses or who are persistently difficult to wean off treatment should have their diagnosis reconsidered. In cases where there is diagnostic uncertainty, refer before starting steroids – there is no urgency for treatment unless there is concern that the patient may have giant cell arteritis.

6. Look for an underlying cause in a patient presenting with Raynaud's phenomenon

Primary Raynaud's usually starts in adolescence or early adulthood, and often runs in families. Less often, Raynaud's phenomenon may be secondary to occupation (as in drill users) or drugs such as beta-blockers. Alternatively, there may be an underlying connective tissue disease. Look for features of lupus, scleroderma or inflammatory arthritis. New onset Raynaud's phenomenon in an older male is rare – if this occurs, consider malignancy. Patients in whom there could be an underlying cause should be referred, whereas patients with primary Raynaud's can be managed in the community, as they seldom suffer complications. Advise conservative measures such as wearing gloves and avoiding low-temperature environments. In some cases, calcium channel blockers may be required. The COVID-19 virus has caused a significant increase in chilblains. The lesions can be pruritic, tender and erythematous. They can resemble Raynaud's phenomenon and are treated in a similar way. If there is significant pain and pruritus, a mild topical steroid cream could be helpful to alleviate symptoms, although non-medical measures usually suffice.

7. Check the urine of patients with suspected or established rheumatological disease

In the case of suspected rheumatological disease, microscopic haematuria could represent renal vasculitis or glomerulonephritis (e.g. in ANCA vasculitis or lupus) and often precedes deterioration in the serum creatinine level. Proteinuria can be seen as a result of acute glomerular disease (e.g. lupus nephritis) but also in relation to renal amyloidosis – a consequence of long-standing inflammatory disease. If a rheumatological disorder or flare of a known rheumatological condition is suspected, a urinalysis should always be performed as part of the clinical assessment.

8. Consider steroids to treat a flare of inflammatory arthritis

In patients with inflammatory arthritis who have multiple synovitic joints (and in whom there is no suggestion of sepsis), 120 mg Depo-Medrone® administered intramuscularly or a short course of oral prednisolone (20–30 mg daily, weaning over 4 weeks) will usually be effective in terminating the flare. It is important to inform the treating rheumatologist, as a flare can be a sign of inadequate treatment requiring escalation of therapy.

9. Tailor management of chronic pain syndrome and fibromyalgia, and remain optimistic

These can be some of the most challenging conditions for both patients and doctors to manage. Fibromyalgia can be a patient's primary rheumatological diagnosis or occur in association with another condition such as inflammatory arthritis or lupus. Optimal management of chronic pain usually involves a three-pronged approach of physiotherapy (graded exercise programme), medication and cognitive behavioural therapy. If medication is needed, the following antidepressants are recommended: amitriptyline, citalopram, duloxetine, fluoxetine or sertraline.

If an antidepressant is offered, explain that it is because these medicines can improve quality of life, pain, sleep and psychological distress, even in the absence of a diagnosis of depression. Pregabalin, gabapentin, opioids and NSAIDs are not recommended. Not all approaches will be wanted or required. It is important that doctors remind patients that chronic pain symptoms can improve, and symptoms often wax and wane.

10. Remember the possibility of significant rheumatological disease in children

Inflammatory arthritis, lupus and other connective tissue diseases can occur in children and adolescents. However, these patients may not be forthcoming about their symptoms, so it is important to ask specifically about key symptoms such as joint pain and swelling, rashes, Raynaud's, sicca symptoms, and other constitutional symptoms such as weight loss, malaise and anorexia. Patients may have given up activities they normally enjoy or become more withdrawn, and teachers may have noticed a deterioration in educational performance. These diseases require careful clinical examination. A urine dipstick may reveal early evidence of nephritis. Do not hesitate to refer for a specialist opinion if in doubt. Systemic lupus erythematosus (SLE) in children can be more aggressive, with a higher incidence of renal disease.

Obscure or Overlooked Diagnoses

1. Hypermobility syndrome

Hypermobility syndrome is defined as 'musculoskeletal symptoms in the presence of generalised joint laxity in otherwise normal subjects'. It is more common in females and younger people. It can be seen as part of an inherited connective tissue disorder, such as Ehlers–Danlos syndrome, or, more commonly, in patients without such a disorder. Patients may present with arthralgia or a history of recurrent joint subluxation or dislocation. Without a diagnosis or appropriate interventions, over time, musculoskeletal symptoms may evolve into a chronic pain syndrome. Specialist physiotherapy and cognitive behavioural therapy can be effective. The Beighton Score is used in clinical practice to assess for hypermobility.

2. RS3PE

Remitting seronegative symmetrical synovitis with pitting oedema (RS3PE) is characterised by bilateral swelling of the hands and/or feet with marked pitting oedema. Patients are often older, with a male preponderance, and tests for rheumatoid factor and anti-CCP antibody are negative. Inflammatory markers are raised. There is an association with malignancy, so further investigations are recommended. In the absence of malignancy, this disease typically responds well to low-dose steroids and remits.

3. SAPHO

This is a syndrome characterised by synovitis, acne, pustulosis, hyperostosis and osteitis. The synovitis usually presents as a large joint oligoarticular arthritis involving the hip, knee, ankle or sacroiliac joints. Osteitis most commonly occurs in the clavicle and may cause arthritis at the articulation with the sternum or the ribs. Chronic inflammation leads to hyperostosis, most often seen in the sternoclavicular joints. Patients may have severe acne or palmoplantar pustulosis (PPP).

There is some dispute as to whether SAPHO represents a subset of seronegative spondyloarthropathies. Treatment of the acne is usually in conjunction with a dermatologist, but the bone and joint manifestations can be treated with disease-modifying antirheumatic drugs.

Easily Confused

1. Septic arthritis and gout

	Septic arthritis	*Gout*
History	■ Risk factors: immunosuppression, diabetes, recent joint instrumentation, sepsis elsewhere, portal of entry	■ Possible previous episodes of gout, or known hyperuricaemia ■ Risk factors: excess alcohol, high purine diet, renal impairment, obesity, diuretics
Examination	■ Clinical features of sepsis: fever, may appear constitutionally unwell ■ Reduced range of movement of the joint which is swollen, hot and tender	■ Gouty tophi may be present ■ Patients may have a low-grade temperature; not normally constitutionally unwell ■ If affected joint is the first metatarsophalangeal joint (MTPJ), this is likely to be acute gout ■ Range of movement is also reduced in acute gout and it can be as painful as septic arthritis
Investigations	■ Blood cultures may be positive ■ Joint aspiration yields synovial fluid with positive gram stain, growth or polymerase chain reaction for bacterial DNA, though if antibiotics are administered prior to aspiration, culture may be negative	■ History of hyperuricaemia on previous blood testing ■ Uric acid may be normal/low in acute episode ■ Radiograph may show evidence of 'punched out' gouty erosions from previous episodes ■ Joint aspiration yields synovial fluid with crystals seen under polarised light microscopy, although negative microscopy does not exclude gout

2. SLE and fibromyalgia

	SLE	*Fibromyalgia*
History	■ Some of the clinical features of SLE and fibromyalgia overlap, such as fatigue, arthralgia and myalgia ■ Patients report multisystem problems: photosensitive rash, mouth ulcers, sicca symptoms, Raynaud's phenomenon, pleuritic chest pain, fever, alopecia and weight loss ■ In the case of secondary antiphospholipid syndrome, there may be a history of recurrent venous or arterial thromboembolism, or miscarriage	■ No other classical SLE symptoms
Examination	■ *Evidence of features as above plus:* ■ Lymphadenopathy or splenomegaly ■ Nail fold abnormalities ■ Reduced salivary pool ■ Jaccoud's arthropathy ■ Pleural or pericardial rub ■ Peripheral oedema may be present if there is severe renal involvement	■ Joint or muscle tenderness may be present, but no arthropathy or true weakness ■ It can be difficult to differentiate between weakness and pain
Investigations	■ Possible proteinuria/microscopic haematuria ■ Raised ESR (and CRP if serositis/arthritis is present) ■ Anaemia, lymphopenia, thrombocytopenia ■ Positive ANA in 95% cases, high titre is more specific ■ Positive ENA/dsDNA and antiphospholipid antibodies ■ Low complement may occur	■ Normal urine dip ■ Normal blood tests including a weak positive ANA which is a common, normal finding

3. Temporal arteritis and tension headaches

	Temporal arteritis	*Tension headaches*
History	■ Most common in older patients (aged 60 years and above) ■ New headache, which may be unilateral or bilateral ■ Visual disturbance ■ Jaw claudication ■ Scalp pain on hair brushing ■ Fever, malaise and weight loss may be present ■ Overlap with symptoms of polymyalgia rheumatica	■ No visual disturbance, jaw claudication or constitutional symptoms ■ May be associated with stress ■ A band-like, 'tight' ache of moderate intensity ■ Fronto-occipital distribution common ■ Usually responds to over-the-counter analgesia

(Continued)

Examination	■ Patient may be systemically unwell ■ Scalp tenderness most marked along the course of the extracranial arteries ■ Temporal artery may be thickened with loss of pulsation ■ Loss of visual acuity, abnormal pupillary reflexes, diplopia, cranial nerve palsies ■ Pallor of the optic disc	■ Tenderness may be present over the scalp or neck, but not particularly localised to the artery
Investigations	■ Elevated ESR for age and CRP, but note inflammatory markers can occasionally be normal ■ Temporal artery ultrasound can show a thickened vessel wall ('halo sign') ■ PET-CT can show active vessel wall inflammation, i.e. aorta, subclavian, vertebral arteries ■ Temporal artery biopsy shows evidence of giant cells in the arterial wall	■ Normal ESR for age ■ Normal CRP

Prescribing Points

1. **Steroids**

   Remember that, to prevent an Addisonian crisis, patients on long-term steroids who become acutely unwell or undergo surgery must double their steroid dose until the acute illness has subsided.

2. **Allopurinol**

   Do not stop this drug during an acute flare of gout. Simply treat the acute attack with either an NSAID, a short course of prednisolone or colchicine 500 mcg two to three times a day. When increasing the dose of allopurinol once the flare has settled or when starting it for the first time, cover the patient with colchicine 500 mcg twice a day to prevent flares for up to 6 months. The recommended target urate level is <300 mmol/L (5 mg/dL).

3. **Methotrexate**

   If the patient has an infection, withhold the methotrexate until the infection has been fully treated and the patient has recovered. In the case of urinary tract infections, do not give trimethoprim – the combination with recent methotrexate causes bone marrow suppression.

4. Biologic therapy

Biologic therapies (often called 'biologics') are now the standard of care for many rheumatic diseases, each designed to target an inflammatory cytokine in order to disrupt the inflammatory cascade and cycle of inflammation. New molecular targets and associated drugs are being developed year on year. Although these drugs have revolutionised the care of patients with rheumatic disease, they are not without risk and require close monitoring of patients. Biologics are prescribed in secondary/tertiary care.

Opportunistic infections, including *Pneumocystis* pneumonia (PCP) and tuberculosis (TB), are more common in patients on immunosuppressive

Table 28.1 Biologics in autoimmune rheumatic disease

Biologic	Indication	Pitfalls
TNF inhibition: i.e. etanercept, adalimumab, golimumab, certolizumab, infliximab	Rheumatoid arthritis, psoriatic arthritis, ankylosing spondylitis	Reactivation of, or *de novo*, tuberculosis (TB). If a patient on TNF inhibitor presents with a febrile illness which does not respond to typical antibiotics, consider TB.
B-cell targeted: rituximab, belimumab	SLE, ANCA-associated vasculitis, rheumatoid arthritis	For rituximab, ideally vaccinations should be timed 4 weeks before the next cycle of treatment is due in order to maximise a patient's chance of producing a good vaccine response. This may not always be possible, dependent on disease activity and patient preferences. Rituximab may cause hypogammaglobulinaemia. Repeated infections should trigger a check of immunoglobulin levels, though these should be repeated by the patient's rheumatologist before and after each cycle of treatment.
Interleukin inhibitors		
IL-6 Tocilizumab/ sarilumab	Rheumatoid arthritis, giant cell arteritis	Normalises CRP and ESR. Retain a high index of suspicion for infection
IL-17 Secukinumab Ixekizumab IL-12/23 Ustekinumab	Psoriatic arthritis	Nasopharyngitis, diarrhoea, upper respiratory tract infections
IL-1 Anakinra	Stills, HLH	Neutropaenia
JAK inhibitors Tofacitinib Baricitinib Upadacitinib Filgotinib	Rheumatoid arthritis, psoriatic arthritis	Herpes zoster, increased risk of VTE
T-cell inhibitors Abatacept	Rheumatoid arthritis	Mild chest or urinary infections

Table 28.2 Abnormal laboratory parameters in DMARD monitoring

Blood test	Value
White cell count	$<3.5 \times 10^9/L$
Neutrophil	$<1.6 \times 10^9/L$
Mean cell volume (MCV)	>105 fL
Platelet count	$<140 \times 10^9/L$
Eosinophilia	$>0.5 \times 10^9/L$
Creatinine/eGFR	Increase in creatinine $>30\%$ from baseline
ALT and/or AST	>100 IU/L
Albumin	<30 g/L

therapies, particularly biologics. Be aware that patients may not present with typical features of infection (i.e. fever, rise in CRP), and a high index of suspicion needs to be maintained.

Table 28.1 categorises the most commonly used biologic medications in autoimmune rheumatic disease, their primary indication and common pitfalls to be aware of when managing patients on these medications.

5. **Pregnancy**

Hydroxychloroquine, sulfasalazine and azathioprine can be continued during pregnancy, but many others should be avoided and/or discussed with a rheumatologist. NSAIDs should be avoided in the third trimester. Prednisolone should be considered for use during pregnancy if it is required to control active disease.

6. **Disease-modifying anti-rheumatic drugs (DMARDs) – monitoring and shared care agreements**

The responsibility of DMARD prescribing and monitoring lies with the rheumatologist until the patient is on a stable dose. Initial monitoring includes FBC, creatinine/calculated GFR, ALT and/or AST, and albumin every 2 weeks until on a stable dose for 6 weeks; then once on a stable dose, monthly FBC, creatinine/calculated GFR, ALT and/or AST, and albumin for 3 months; thereafter, FBC, creatinine/calculated GFR, ALT and/or AST, and albumin at least every 12 weeks. Dose increases should be monitored every 2 weeks for 6 weeks until on a stable dose and then revert to the previous schedule. It is common practice, once the patient is established on their medication (usually by 6 months), that further prescriptions and blood test monitoring are undertaken in primary care with guidance in the form of a shared care agreement. Table 28.2 shows parameters for blood test values that should prompt discussion with your local rheumatology team and consideration of interruption in treatment. As well as absolute values, trends in results should also be observed, and if any concern, early discussion with your local rheumatology team is advised.

SEXUAL HEALTH

Michael Rayment

Ten Pearls of Wisdom

1. Be proactive about HIV testing

People living with HIV can anticipate a normal life expectancy if they are diagnosed with a CD4 count >350 cells/μL and have access to antiretroviral therapy (ART). Achieving an undetectable viral load with ART also eliminates the risk of onward transmission of the virus ('undetectable = untransmittable' or 'U = U'). Despite this, about 40% of people with HIV infection in the UK are diagnosed late (with counts <350 cells/μL) and around a tenth do not know their positive status. The gateway to HIV treatment and prevention is HIV testing, including in primary care. Offer a test to anyone in a demographic risk group, with a sexually transmitted infection (STI), with an HIV 'indicator disease' (like viral hepatitis) or with features of immunosuppression. In high-prevalence areas (a prevalence of 2/1000 persons or more), offer a test to all new registrants, and in areas of extremely high prevalence (greater than 5/1000 persons) offer a test to everyone having a blood test for any indication. It is in everyone's interest to know their HIV status. Lengthy HIV pre-test counselling belongs to a time before antiretroviral therapy.

2. Do not underestimate erectile dysfunction – it may herald coronary artery disease

Various studies demonstrate a link between erectile dysfunction (ED) and coronary heart disease (CHD). In patients with moderate to severe ED, the relative risk of CHD in 10 years is 14% in men aged 30–39 years old and up to 27% in men over 60 years old. The narrow bore of the cavernosal arteries relative to the coronaries may explain the presentation of vascular ED before CHD. All men with ED should have a cardiovascular risk assessment, risk reduction advice and primary prevention interventions, as appropriate. In men at high risk or with poor exercise tolerance, consider stress testing, coronary calcium scoring or referral to cardiology.

3. Know your local STI epidemiology

The epidemiology of STIs is unique among infectious diseases in that it is significantly influenced by demography; behavioural and attitudinal change; socioeconomic factors; drug, alcohol and substance use; and testing patterns

DOI: 10.1201/9781003304586-29

and access to online and in-person services. The UK has some of the most complete STI surveillance in the world, and the data paint a picture of extremes from urban to rural, from affluence to deprivation. Learn about your local epidemiology (https://fingertips.phe.org.uk/profile/sexualhealth/data) so you can be equipped to help address sexual ill health.

4. Consider pelvic inflammatory disease in all sexually active women with subacute pelvic pain

Pelvic inflammatory disease (PID) has a few unique signs and symptoms. Subacute lower abdominal pain and deep dyspareunia are suggestive, with or without vaginal discharge and unscheduled bleeding. Cervical excitation is a relatively specific sign, and adnexal tenderness, if present, will usually be bilateral. Risk factors for PID include younger age (less than 25 years), a new sexual partner, more than three lifetime sexual partners and a history of STI. Use of hormonal contraception reduces risk (especially progesterone-only methods) and PID is very rare in second- and third-trimester pregnancy. Approximately 10%–30% of cases of untreated *Chlamydia trachomatis* (CT) and *Neisseria gonorrhoeae* (NG) cervicitis proceed to PID – as a minimum, swabs should be taken for these pathogens. However, no organism is isolated in most cases. Antimicrobial treatment reduces the risk of sequelae (such as tubal factor infertility and chronic pelvic pain).

5. If you don't ask the question, you won't hear the answer

Taking a sexual history enables us to undertake an STI risk assessment; enquire about sexual difficulties; and offer screening, intervention and referral. People may have sexual health needs at various life stages (e.g. during mental illness, after surgery, during menopause, after myocardial infarction) and a failure to discuss sex alongside other aspects of health is a missed opportunity. It is helpful to normalise sex and enquiries relating to it (e.g. 'Lots of men are worried about having sex again after a heart attack. How are you feeling about it?'). Agree on a common vocabulary but do not use language that makes you feel uncomfortable. Stick to the facts and not the values.

6. A copper intra-uterine device is the most effective method of emergency contraception and can be used late in the cycle, after multiple episodes of unprotected sex

Studies demonstrate that the copper intra-uterine device (IUD) is not offered enough to women requesting emergency contraception, despite being the most effective method. Reasons are manifold but often include operational factors (e.g. a lack of skilled personnel and time) and attitudinal factors about acceptability (usually on the side of the clinician). Importantly, the IUD has both pre- and post-fertilisation effects (it acts as a spermicide, ovicide and prevents implantation). Thus, if the woman is appropriately counselled on a possible post-fertilisation effect, an IUD can be used up to 5 days after the patient's earliest expected date of ovulation, even if multiple episodes of sex have taken place since the last menstrual period.

7. Try to find the cause in men with urethritis

Men with features of acute urethritis (dysuria, and/or urethral discharge) are presenting with a syndrome with multiple possible infectious and non-infectious causes. Lower urinary tract symptoms other than dysuria suggest an alternative diagnosis. No signs or symptoms can reliably discriminate one infectious cause from another without diagnostics (such as gram staining, culture or nucleic acid amplification testing [NAAT]). In the surgery, a urinalysis of first-void urine can be undertaken. If this shows leucocytes only, urethritis is likely. Send NAAT for CT/NG as a minimum. First-line empirical treatment should be with doxycycline. It will treat CT–urethritis, and 50% of cases of *Mycoplasma genitalium* urethritis. It is probably better to refer all men to a sexual health clinic, and always refer if there is copious purulent discharge (suggesting gonococcal urethritis).

8. When diagnosing one STI, screen for others

Increasingly, STI screens are performed outside sexual health clinics, which is progress. The more tests that are done, the more cases of STI – such as CT – are found and treated, breaking chains of infection. However, the presence of one STI increases the likelihood of others. For example, 10% of people with first presentation of anogenital warts will have a co-existent STI. So, if you diagnose an STI, screen for others (as per British Association for Sexual Health and HIV standards [www.bashh.org]) or refer the patient to a sexual health clinic.

9. The most common cause of vaginal discharge is bacterial vaginosis, not candidiasis

Vaginal discharge is the most common presentation to sexual health clinics, and patients present very commonly to primary care, too. Ask about the colour, consistency and odour of the discharge. Ask about exacerbating factors, such as menses, sex or hygiene products and practices. Most importantly, ask about inflammatory symptoms such as itch and superficial dyspareunia (see the 'Easily confused' section). Based on history alone, it is possible to make a fairly confident diagnosis, and it is reasonable to give one course of treatment on an empirical basis. All women with atypical features, or those whose symptoms persist or recur following treatment, should have a vulval and speculum examination.

10. Don't forget the partner!

STIs affect more than the patient in front of you. If you refer a patient to a sexual health clinic, suggest that their partner goes too. If treating STIs in primary care, remember partner notification and their need for screening and/or treatment. Your patient will likely be prepared to talk to their partners themselves, assuaging confidentiality concerns. If they think this will be a challenge, refer to sexual health where other methods of partner notification can be undertaken (such as direct contact, or online and mobile SMS methods). Partners may be treated for the infection of concern on attendance, in addition to being screened.

Obscure and Overlooked Diagnoses

1. **Lymphogranuloma venereum**

   Once a rare infection in the UK, *Lymphogranuloma venereum* (LGV) is a syndrome caused by invasive serovars of CT. Since 2004, cases have been reported in men who have sex with men, and now we see about 1,000 cases per year. Men present with subacute rectal symptoms (including discharge and tenesmus) and sometimes with systemic features such as malaise and weight loss, mimicking inflammatory bowel disease (IBD). Treatment is with prolonged doxycycline. Take a sexual history, and in all men who have sex with men with proctitic symptoms, test for the infection with a rectal swab for CT. If positive for CT, refer to the local sexual health service.

2. **Vestibulodynia**

   Vestibulodynia is a relatively common condition characterised by hypersensitivity of light touch to the vestibule, experienced at penetration by intercourse or tampon insertion. There may be secondary vaginismus and there may be erythema at the vestibule. Gentle application of pressure with a cotton swab at the introitus may reproduce the pain, which is always out of proportion to the stimulus. Explaining the reality of the condition can really help. Try 5% lignocaine ointment applied to the vestibule on a cotton bud 15 minutes before penetration. Low-dose amitriptyline may also be helpful. Refer, if necessary, to a sexual health or vulval clinic, or to the Vulval Pain Society online.

3. **Secondary syphilis**

   The incidence of syphilis in the UK has been increasing for several years. Males account for 94% of all diagnoses (the majority being men who have sex with men). Secondary syphilis arises in about 30% of patients, 6 weeks to 6 months after infection. It is a multisystem disorder, and patients with clinical manifestations (e.g. rash, lymphadenopathy, glomerulonephritis, cranial nerve palsies and alopecia) will present to all healthcare providers. Undertake a sexual health risk assessment, offer testing and refer to a sexual health clinic if tests are positive.

4. **Lichen nitidus**

   This has unknown aetiology and presents in children and young adults as a rash characterised by flesh-coloured papules, 1–2 mm in diameter. The glans penis is a common site, as is the chest and the flexor aspects of the wrists and forearms.

Koebnerisation is common. It can look a little like molluscum contagiosum, but the papules lack the typical umbilicus. Treatment is usually conservative, but topical steroids may be helpful if itchy. It will resolve after a variable period of time.

Easily Confused

1. Lichen planus (LP) and lichen sclerosus

Lichen planus (LP)	Lichen sclerosus
■ Variable appearance (papulosquamous [classical], erosive, hypertrophic) ■ Affects squamous skin and mucous membranes; erosive variants often affect vagina. Look for lacy-white edges ■ Extragenital manifestations common (wrists, mouth, gums) ■ Itch is common, but may be asymptomatic; erosive variant is usually painful ■ Moderate to potent topical steroids often work; erosive LP can be challenging to treat; stop drugs that might be implicated (thiazides, beta-blockers, NSAIDs)	■ Atrophic, 'ivory-white' appearance with local, involutional architectural destruction ■ Anogenital 'figure of 8' distribution ■ Extragenital manifestations rare (<10%; may involve back, wrists and sub-mammary areas) ■ Itch is predominant, and secondary symptoms from architectural change (e.g. dyspareunia in women, splitting of frenulum in men) ■ Responds to very potent topical steroids

2. Bacterial vaginosis and vulvovaginal candidiasis

Bacterial vaginosis	Vulvovaginal candidiasis
■ Homogeneous, grey-white discharge, usually with an offensive smell (often worse after sex or menstruation) ■ No inflammatory symptoms ■ Vulval examination normal, but vagina demonstrates homogeneous discharge; pH >4.5 on strip testing	■ Non-offensive white discharge, usually 'cottage cheese' type but may be watery ■ Acute vulvovaginitis, with itch, redness, swelling, superficial dyspareunia ■ Vulval erythema, satellite lesions, vaginitis, non-offensive clumpy discharge; culture usually positive (but beware Candida sp. commensal in 20%)

3. Anogenital herpes simplex and anogenital aphthous ulceration

Anogenital herpes simplex	Anogenital aphthous ulceration
■ The most common cause of genital ulceration in the UK ■ Acute vesicular eruption – in crops or more diffuse vesicles quickly de-roof and become painful ulcers ■ Systemic features common in primary episode, with regional, tender lymphadenopathy	■ Usually a diagnosis of exclusion, with patients typically having multiple episodes before diagnosis ■ Variable appearance, but usually acute, atraumatic ulcers that are shallow, single and may be large; recurrent; usually history of oral ulceration ■ Systemic features and prodrome rare (unless a feature of Behcet's disease)

Prescribing Points

1. **Be mindful of drug interactions in patients on antiretroviral therapy**
   ART can cause several interactions with other medications. HIV services have worked hard in recent years to increase communication with primary care, and most patients will consent to correspondence with their GP. If you have not heard from the HIV clinic in a while, demand to know why. ART remains exclusively dispensed from hospitals, so make sure you record co-prescribed ART on the patient's record. The class of ART with the most clinically important drug interactions are protease inhibitors, which are invariably 'boosted' with low doses of ritonavir or cobicistat, both potent inhibitors (and sometimes inducers) of cytochrome P450 enzymes. If a drug is metabolised via the liver, chances are ritonavir and/or cobicistat will affect it. Interactions may range from trivial to life-threatening. Ritonavir should not be given with simvastatin, for example, as simvastatin levels can rise substantially, increasing the risk of rhabdomyolysis. Newer classes of ART, such as integrase inhibitors (raltegravir, dolutegravir) have far fewer effects. A useful, freely accessible resource is available at www.hiv-druginteractions.org, maintained by the University of Liverpool.

2. **Psychotropic medication and sexual side effects**
   Counsel patients on the sexual side effects of psychotropic medication before initiation. Effects include retarded ejaculation, erectile dysfunction and reduced libido. Many patients will not volunteer such side effects without direct enquiry, and within-class changes (e.g. from paroxetine to citalopram in the case of retarded ejaculation) can help.

3. **Treating chlamydia in pregnancy**
   CT infection in pregnancy can be safely treated with azithromycin. Although the summary of product characteristics of azithromycin states that there are insufficient data to support its use, clinical experience and published studies suggest azithromycin is safe and effective. UK guidelines and the WHO recommend first-line use of azithromycin in pregnant women.

4. **Quick start contraception in women at risk of unplanned pregnancy**
   'Quick start' contraception means starting a method without waiting for the next menstrual period. It is safe, easy and reduces the risk of unplanned pregnancy. Offer a 'quick start method' to a woman requesting emergency contraception if you can be reasonably sure she is not already pregnant. If she desires a long-acting method, a 'bridging' short-acting method, such as the combined pill or the progesterone-only pill, can be used until pregnancy can be reliably excluded.

5. **HIV pre-exposure prophylaxis is safe and effective**
   HIV pre-exposure prophylaxis (PrEP) refers to the use of antiretroviral medication by HIV-negative people to reduce their risk of HIV acquisition. The most commonly studied medication is a fixed-dose combination of emtricitabine

and tenofovir, which has been shown to reduce the risk of infection by >90% when taken daily or 'on demand'. It is safe and well tolerated and is almost certainly a cost-effective intervention. PrEP, alongside frequent HIV testing and ART, has resulted in marked reductions in new HIV diagnoses in the UK. PrEP is widely available on the NHS via sexual health clinics across the UK. The biggest user group is men who have sex with men, but other populations (such as trans people, people who inject drugs or heterosexuals belonging to higher-risk groups) may benefit from PrEP. PrEP confers no protection against other STIs. Refer patients to the local sexual health clinic for advice, supply and monitoring.

6. **HIV post-exposure prophylaxis: risk assessment and timely initiation are key**

HIV post-exposure prophylaxis (PEP) remains an important emergency intervention for people exposed to HIV after sexual and non-sexual exposure. It consists of a 28-day course of raltegravir, plus emtricitabine/tenofovir and is well tolerated with few drug interaction considerations. In the era of U = U, sex with a person living with HIV who is undetectable on treatment does not indicate a need for PEP – in fact, it is statistically the safest sex of all as regards HIV transmission! The risk of HIV acquisition depends on who the patient has had sex with, and the kind of sex they have had. A risk assessment is key. If PEP is indicated, timely initiation is important, and PEP must always be commenced within 72 hours of exposure. Community needlestick injuries never indicate a need for PEP (but remember hepatitis B vaccination and follow-up hepatitis C testing) and rarely do bite or spitting attacks require PEP. Check out BASHH guidance online. If in doubt, refer to sexual health or the emergency department.

THYROID DISORDERS

Mark P.J. Vanderpump

Ten Pearls of Wisdom

1. A normal thyroid-stimulating hormone (TSH) excludes primary hypothyroidism

The diagnosis of primary hypothyroidism is based on clinical features supported by biochemical evidence of elevated serum TSH, and low or normal free thyroxine (T4). Because the symptoms of hypothyroidism overlap with those of a variety of chronic disease states, primary hypothyroidism should not be diagnosed based on symptoms alone in individuals with a normal serum TSH. Such practice may lead to an erroneous label of hypothyroidism in a person with another condition and will ultimately result in dissatisfaction with levothyroxine (L-T4) therapy. UK national audit data suggest that over 10% of those started on L-T4 in primary care initially had a normal serum TSH.

2. A significant minority of patients on L-T4 have ongoing symptoms despite 'normal' thyroid function tests

Non-specific symptoms such as lethargy, 'brain fog' and difficulty with weight management occur in up to 5%–10% of people treated for hypothyroidism with a serum TSH within the reference range. Symptoms such as tiredness may have been initially misattributed to hypothyroidism (when in fact they may, for example, have been caused by a mood disorder) with relatively minor biochemical abnormalities found coincidentally during diagnostic work-up with blood screening. Other explanations include awareness of having a chronic disease, adjustment to being euthyroid – particularly in those recently treated for hyperthyroidism – and autoimmunity. Relative risks of almost all other autoimmune diseases are significantly increased (rheumatoid arthritis, pernicious anaemia, systemic lupus erythematosus, Addison's disease, coeliac disease, myasthenia gravis and vitiligo). Screening for other autoimmune diseases is recommended in those presenting with new or non-specific symptoms.

DOI: 10.1201/9781003304586-30

3. Measurement of serum triiodothyronine (T3) is of no value in hypothyroidism

Serum triiodothyronine (T3) levels can remain within the reference range even in severe hypothyroidism. The measurement of T3 is not recommended or required for the diagnosis of hypothyroidism or for the monitoring of thyroid hormone replacement in known hypothyroidism, as its value remains to be ascertained. Serum TSH remains the key biochemical indicator of thyroid function reflecting T4 to T3 conversion and T3 action, so pituitary TSH secretion remains the most sensitive indicator of thyroid status.

4. Ensure consistent L-T4 administration if recurrent abnormal serum TSH levels

People previously stable on long-term L-T4 replacement, those with persistently abnormal serum TSH levels should be reviewed to ensure that L-T4 is being taken correctly. Preferably L-T4 should be administered with water on an empty stomach at least 30 minutes before breakfast and avoiding other medication, especially iron supplements and calcium salts. Disease states that interfere with L-T4 absorption include coeliac disease, pernicious anaemia, gastritis or malabsorption. Rarely, Addison's disease can present as a sudden rise in serum TSH. A raised free T4 and raised serum TSH can be seen in a patient poorly compliant with L-T4 who recommences L-T4 treatment shortly before a blood test. Also, bear in mind that, preferably, thyroid function tests should be performed at the same time of day each time, as there is a diurnal variation in serum TSH levels.

5. Treat subclinical hypothyroidism if serum TSH >10 mU/L or positive thyroid antibodies

Subclinical hypothyroidism is defined as a raised serum TSH and normal T4 and T3 levels. Treatment is generally advised in people with positive thyroid antibodies (usually thyroid peroxidase antibodies [TPOAb]) or serum TSH >10 mU/L, as progression to overt hypothyroidism is more likely in such individuals. Younger persons (<65 years old) with cardiovascular risk factors should also be treated, since studies have shown an association between subclinical hypothyroidism and cardiovascular mortality. It is also reasonable to treat those with goitre or symptoms suggesting hypothyroidism, and women who are pregnant or intending conception because of the potential risk of adverse pregnancy outcomes. If treatment is not advised, monitoring of serum TSH should be carried out 6–12 monthly.

6. A wait-and-see approach is reasonable in subclinical hyperthyroidism

Subclinical hyperthyroidism is defined as a low serum TSH but normal T4 and T3 and has a prevalence of 1%. Elderly people and those with cardiovascular disease are at increased risk of atrial fibrillation; increased bone loss is also reported. If the serum TSH is between 0.1 and 0.4 mU/L, the risk of progression to overt hyperthyroidism is negligible and there are no significant end-organ effects. But if the serum TSH is persistently undetectable (<0.1 mU/L), an endocrine assessment is needed to establish the aetiology and for possible treatment. For most, adopting a wait-and-see approach is appropriate with monitoring of free T4, free T3 and TSH every 6 to 12 months. If the free T3 alone is raised, this is termed 'T3 toxicosis', and should be managed as for overt hyperthyroidism.

7. Hyperthyroidism is not a diagnosis – it is important to establish the cause

Hyperthyroidism commonly results from Graves' disease, toxic multinodular goitre or toxic nodule. Drug causes include amiodarone, lithium and ingestion of products containing high iodine loads. Transient causes include viral and silent autoimmune thyroiditis, which cause self-limiting thyrotoxicosis due to the release of preformed hormones from a damaged thyroid gland, rather than overproduction of thyroid hormones. High-dose biotin supplements can result in spurious hyperthyroidism including positive TSH receptor antibodies (TSHRAb). There are often clues in the history (family history, recent pregnancy, pain and tenderness over the thyroid, drugs) and clinical signs (presence of orbitopathy, smooth or nodular goitre). CRP or ESR is elevated in cases of viral thyroiditis. The TSHRAb assays have a greater than 95% sensitivity and specificity for Graves' disease. A positive TPOAb indicates autoimmune thyroid disease but is not diagnostic and can be found in both transient autoimmune thyroiditis and the persisting hyperthyroidism of Graves' disease.

8. Consider initiating treatment of hyperthyroidism in primary care

Antithyroid treatment with carbimazole or propylthiouracil (PTU) ('thionamides') can be initiated in primary care after discussion with the endocrine team, pending hospital appointment. Beta-blockers such as propranolol should be considered for symptomatic relief and can be safely initiated in most cases of hyperthyroidism unless there is a history of asthma. They can provide relief of anxiety, tremor and palpitation, and can help protect the heart against arrhythmia. Initiation of treatment in primary care is particularly relevant in severe clinical or biochemical hyperthyroidism, in elderly people, or in those with known cardiac problems or arrhythmia – particularly if there is likely to be delay in getting the person seen in the hospital clinic.

9. Graves' orbitopathy (GO) may precede hyperthyroidism

Early symptoms of GO include grittiness, photophobia, lacrimation, swelling and redness of the eyelids and conjunctiva, restriction of eye movements, double or blurred vision, or retro-orbital pain. There may not always be significant exophthalmos. Although usually a clinical diagnosis, the TSHRAb will typically be positive. GO is present in about 50% of people with Graves' disease and is severe and potentially sight-threatening in 3%–5%. In most cases, GO and hyperthyroidism occur within 18 months of each other, although GO may precede or follow the onset of hyperthyroidism. In approximately 5%, no evidence of hyperthyroidism is found (dysthyroid eye disease) – and GO can be unilateral. It may also rarely occur in Hashimoto's thyroiditis. Stopping smoking, controlling thyroid dysfunction, selenium supplements and eye lubricants are beneficial. Specialist assessment is required to consider MRI if there is diagnostic doubt and to assess whether glucocorticoids or immunosuppression are required.

10. Avoid indiscriminate ultrasound imaging of the thyroid

Although benign thyroid nodules are common, thyroid cancers are rare (annual incidence 2–3 per 100,000 population). Thyroid cancer incidence has increased due to the increased detection of clinically silent papillary microcarcinomas (diameter <1 cm) which have been reported in 10% of adults at post-mortem. Ultrasonography as a screening tool is too sensitive and will result in the unnecessary pursuit of findings that are common and rarely have pathological significance. It may have a place in investigating people presenting with thyroid nodules to determine whether they are single or multiple, to provide an accurate indication of thyroid size and to differentiate cystic nodules from solid ones. Consider a suspected cancer pathway referral for any unexplained thyroid lump, a history of a recent increase in size, obstructive symptoms, voice changes or associated lymphadenopathy.

Obscure or Overlooked Diagnoses

1. Subacute (viral, de Quervain's) thyroiditis

This is a painful, destructive thyroiditis characterised by hyperthyroidism due to the release of pre-formed hormones. There is usually a preceding viral illness, acute neck pain often radiating to the ear and raised inflammatory markers. The duration of hyperthyroidism is generally 1 to 3 months. Hypothyroidism is common after the hyperthyroid phase but reported as permanent in less than 5%. Specific therapy is usually unnecessary during the hyperthyroid phase, although beta-blockers can be helpful. Thionamides are contraindicated; glucocorticoids may decrease the duration of the clinical syndrome if symptoms persist despite paracetamol and non-steroidal anti-inflammatory drug therapy.

2. Amiodarone-induced thyroid dysfunction

Amiodarone structurally closely resembles thyroid hormones and contains about 37% of organic iodine by weight. Approximately 25% develop thyroid dysfunction (either hypo- or hyperthyroidism) after 2 to 3 years of treatment, and this risk increases with higher cumulative doses – so thyroid function should be routinely tested every 6 months. Amiodarone-induced thyrotoxicosis is usually a destructive thyroiditis occurring in an otherwise normal thyroid gland and is often associated with few symptoms. If found, there is no need to stop amiodarone, but an urgent endocrine referral is warranted, as thyroiditis can be responsive to glucocorticoids rather than thionamide therapy. In amiodarone-induced hypothyroidism, continue amiodarone and replace with L-T4 targeting a serum TSH at the upper end of the reference range.

3. **Post-partum thyroiditis**

Thyroid antibodies, particularly TPOAb, occur in 10% of women at 14 weeks of gestation. After delivery, transient, destructive autoimmune thyroiditis occurs between the 12th and 16th week post-partum in 50% of TPOAb-positive women. It presents as a temporary, usually painless, episode of hypothyroidism, occasionally preceded by a short episode of hyperthyroidism. Up to about a quarter of women progress to permanent hypothyroidism within approximately 5 years, particularly those with high antibody titres.

Easily Confused

1. Weird thyroid function tests and causes

Weird thyroid function test	Causes
Free T4/free T3 normal, low TSH	■ Subclinical hyperthyroidism ■ Recent treatment for hyperthyroidism ■ Drugs (e.g. steroids) ■ Non-thyroidal illness
Free T4/free T3 normal, raised TSH	■ Subclinical hypothyroidism ■ Poor compliance with L-T4 ■ L-T4 malabsorption ■ Drugs (e.g. amiodarone) ■ Assay interference ■ Non-thyroidal illness recovery phase
Free T4/free T3 low, low/normal TSH	■ Non-thyroidal illness ■ Hypopituitarism ■ Isolated TSH deficiency
Free T4/free T3 raised, raised/normal TSH	■ Assay interference ■ L-T4 replacement therapy including poor compliance ■ Drugs (e.g. amiodarone, heparin) ■ Non-thyroidal illness including acute psychiatric disorders ■ Neonatal period ■ TSH-secreting pituitary adenoma ■ Thyroid hormone resistance ■ Thyroid hormone metabolic disorder

2. Primary hypothyroidism and hypopituitarism

Primary hypothyroidism	Hypopituitarism
■ Low FT4	■ Low FT4
■ Raised serum TSH	■ Low/inappropriately normal serum TSH
■ Autoimmune in aetiology with positive thyroid antibodies and family history	■ Usually due to non-functioning pituitary tumour or post pituitary surgery
■ Rare presentation of Addison's disease (primary hypoadrenalism)	■ Biochemical evidence of secondary hypogonadism and hypoadrenalism

3. Increasing suspicion of malignancy and favouring a benign goitre

Increasing suspicion of malignancy	Favouring a benign goitre
■ Age <20 or >50 years old	■ Age 20–50 years old
■ Men	■ Women
■ Mild hypothyroidism	■ Hyperthyroidism
■ Cervical lymphadenopathy	■ Multinodular goitre without dominant nodule
■ Firm, hard, irregular, fixed nodule	■ Soft, smooth, mobile nodule
■ Family history of thyroid cancer	■ Family history of benign thyroid nodule or thyroid autoimmunity
■ History of external neck radiotherapy	■ Associated pain or tenderness
■ Dysphagia/hoarseness/stridor	■ Compression symptoms rare

Prescribing Points

1. **L-T4 and liothyronine (L-T3) combination therapy**

   Evidence from controlled trials has shown no consistent added benefit of combined L-T4 and L-T3 therapy over L-T4 monotherapy in terms of quality of life, mood or psychometric measures. Although some individuals express a preference for combined therapy, there is limited long-term safety data to support its routine use in practice. Specialist referral should be considered in individuals who have unambiguously not benefited from L-T4 and have been thoroughly evaluated for alternative causes of ill health. Animal thyroid desiccated extracts (e.g. 'armour') all have a much higher dose of T3 than is considered physiological and are not recommended.

2. **Side effects of thionamides**

   Although generally well tolerated, agranulocytosis is a rare but potentially fatal side effect occurring in 0.1%–0.5% of cases. As agranulocytosis occurs very suddenly, routine monitoring of full blood count is not recommended. It usually occurs within the first 3 months after initiation of therapy (97% within the first 6 months, especially on higher doses), but cases have occurred a long time after starting treatment. People present with fever and evidence of infection, usually in the oropharynx. Written instructions should be documented as being given to discontinue the medication and check the blood count should the situation arise. Allergic-type reactions of rash, urticaria and arthralgia occur in 1%–5%, are often mild and do not usually necessitate drug withdrawal, although one thionamide may be substituted for another in the expectation that the second agent may be taken without side effects.

3. **Thionamides in pregnancy**

   Thionamides in low dosage can be given relatively safely, and both PTU and carbimazole are effective. Historically, PTU has been preferred, as it is associated with a lower risk of aplasia cutis. However, concern regarding hepatotoxicity of PTU, particularly in children, has led to recommendations that it should only be prescribed pre-conception and in the first trimester, and that carbimazole should be used from the second trimester onwards. The block-replacement regime using a thionamide and L-T4 is contraindicated in pregnant women. Ideally, women should consider definitive treatment of Graves' disease by radioiodine or surgery pre-pregnancy.

4. **L-T4 in pregnancy**

   The dose of L-T4 should be adjusted to ensure that the serum TSH is not higher than 2.5 mU/L prior to conception. In treated hypothyroid women, the serum TSH may rise during pregnancy and they will require an extra 25 to 50 µg daily during the first 4 to 8 weeks of pregnancy to maintain a serum TSH between 0.5 and 2.5 mU/L – especially during the first trimester, as the fetus is completely reliant on maternal thyroid status until the second trimester. Women should be advised to increase their dose of L-T4 by 25 µg as soon as their pregnancy is confirmed. Post-delivery, women should usually be advised to decrease the L-T4 dose to their pre-pregnancy dose.

UROLOGY

Ian Eardley

Ten Pearls of Wisdom

1. Beware recurrent urinary infections in the elderly

Recurrent urinary tract infections (i.e. three or more per year) are a common clinical problem, especially in women, and they are often associated with bleeding. It is important to remember that they can be the presenting feature of bladder cancer – even when there is no visible haematuria, which might otherwise suggest an underlying problem. NICE advises non-urgent referral for investigation of possible bladder cancer in people aged 60 and over with recurrent or persistent unexplained urinary tract infections. Also, those aged 60 or older with dysuria and unexplained non-visible haematuria should be referred urgently, and those aged 45 or older with visible haematuria that persists or recurs after successful treatment of a urinary infection also warrant a cancer pathway referral.

2. Avoid measuring a PSA in urinary retention or after a recent UTI

PSA is an excellent tumour marker for prostate cancer, in that it typically follows the activity of a cancer. However, as a diagnostic test for prostate cancer, it is imperfect and this is particularly so in men who have had a recent urinary tract infection or who have developed urinary retention. PSA testing under these circumstances can be misleading since both conditions will cause an artefactually raised PSA, and this rise can be considerable. So wait until the problem has resolved before arranging the test – given the 2- to 3-day half-life of PSA, a delay of 2 to 3 weeks is necessary before testing.

3. Persistent red patches on the glans penis or prepuce need biopsy

Red skin lesions on the penis are reasonably common, with potential causes ranging from fungal infections to carcinoma *in situ*. The difficulty is in identifying which ones are potentially dangerous. Most inflammatory causes such as a fungal infection will tend to 'come and go', often in response to treatment. Persistent rashes can represent carcinoma *in situ* and are best diagnosed by biopsy, which can be performed under local anaesthetic. Persistence is the single most important feature to look for.

 DOI: 10.1201/9781003304586-31

4. **Sudden onset of bed-wetting in an older man suggests chronic urinary retention, often with renal impairment**

In these men, the bladder is almost always palpable and abdominal examination will detect this. In a more obese man, an ultrasound will identify the enlarged bladder and the hydronephrosis that often accompanies it. Chronic retention of urine in elderly men is usually due to benign prostatic hyperplasia, which causes progressive build-up of urine within the bladder with overflow incontinence, usually at night, that often is not associated with a sensation of bladder fullness. It typically develops gradually over several months and can lead to bilateral hydronephrosis with renal impairment. This problem needs urgent urological referral for catheterisation. When renal function is optimised, the definitive treatment is usually transurethral prostatectomy.

5. **In acute testicular pain, do not be misled by a history of trauma – it could still be torsion**

In a child or young man with a history of acute testicular pain, a co-existent history of trauma should not obscure the potential for the underlying problem to be testicular torsion – the trauma may be coincidental and misattributed by the patient. Testicular torsion is an urgent problem that requires surgical untwisting of the testis within 6 hours if the testis is to be saved. If in doubt, the patient should be referred for urgent surgical assessment.

6. **Ensure any necessary urine specimen is obtained before antibiotics are taken**

Remember that, in a patient with a urinary tract infection, a single dose of an antibiotic can potentially render the urine sterile, with the loss of bacteria from the urine. This will potentially result in false-negative dipsticks (with loss of positivity to nitrites) and urine cultures that demonstrate pyuria but fail to demonstrate growth of bacteria. Try to get the urine specimen for culture before the patient takes any antibiotics to ensure accurate microbiology and appropriate antibiotic use.

7. **Beware of the possibility of cauda equina syndrome in patients who present with acute back pain and recent onset urinary symptoms**

The commonest cause is compression of the cauda equina by a prolapsed intervertebral disc. The received wisdom is that we enquire about urinary incontinence and physical signs involving impaired perineal sensation and reduced anal sphincter tone. But these features are unreliable and when present indicate a late stage of compression – probably too late to repair the damage. Instead, careful history taking should elicit subtle features such as decreased sensation with bladder filling or emptying. If in doubt, refer, even though the majority will turn out to be false alarms – rather this than miss a case. Once urgently referred, the patient needs prompt imaging (typically an MRI) and surgical decompression.

8. Ureteric colic with co-existent fever is a surgical emergency

In a patient who appears to have ureteric colic or who has a known ureteric calculus, the development of fever is potentially serious. It may represent infection within the obstructed system, which can result in pyonephrosis and systemic sepsis, and potentially can be fatal. The patient is often tender in the affected loin. Such cases need urgent referral to hospital where the optimal treatment involves intravenous antibiotics and percutaneous nephrostomy.

9. Clarify what men mean when they present with 'impotence' or 'erectile dysfunction'

The issue may genuinely be erectile dysfunction. But it could also be premature ejaculation (i.e. he gets an erection, but ejaculates too quickly and then loses the erection) or reduced sexual interest – men often use inaccurate terminology for these problems. The basis of diagnosis is a careful clinical history, even if it is sometimes a bit embarrassing for the patient (and perhaps the doctor). Otherwise, the potential outcome is at best confusion and prolonged consultation, or even inappropriate treatment.

10. Beware of a leaking abdominal aortic aneurysm in an older patient with apparent left-sided ureteric colic

Sudden onset loin pain is commonly caused by urological pathologies such as ureteric colic or urinary tract infection. In women, ovarian pathology is another cause, as is musculoskeletal pain. A less common but very significant cause is a leaking abdominal aortic aneurysm, which can present with loin pain that is most commonly left-sided. So, especially if the patient is older and has signs of blood loss, a leaking abdominal aortic aneurysm is a diagnosis to consider.

Obscure and Overlooked Diagnoses

1. Bladder neck obstruction

The commonest cause of lower urinary tract symptoms (LUTS) in older men is enlargement of the prostate, usually due to benign prostatic hyperplasia (BPH). This typically occurs in older men (over 50 years of age) and is characterised by hesitancy, poor urinary stream, frequency of micturition and nocturia. However, a similar set of symptoms can occur in younger men, perhaps as young as 25 years of age. Here, the 'obstruction' is a malfunctioning bladder neck that does not fully relax during micturition and leads to identical urinary symptoms, which may be worse when the man wishes to pass urine 'in public', such as in a public toilet. Treatment is with an alpha-blocker, although a proportion of men will require surgical incision of the bladder neck.

2. **Fowler's syndrome**
   Urinary retention in women is rare. When it happens, causes such as constipation, urinary infection, pelvic masses and neurological disease should be excluded by clinical assessment and if necessary by pelvic ultrasound and MRI of the lumbosacral spine. If these prove negative, then a possible diagnosis is Fowler's syndrome – a rare condition often associated with polycystic ovaries that is idiopathic and associated with a poorly relaxing urethral sphincter. Treatment in the short term is by means of clean intermittent self-catheterisation, but sacral neuromodulation is often a more definitive solution.

3. **Urinary schistosomiasis**
   Painless haematuria in patients who have recently travelled to places such as Egypt or central Africa should raise the possibility of urinary schistosomiasis. This is a parasitic disease contracted when swimming or bathing in infected water where infected freshwater snails release tapeworms, which penetrate people's skin and causes the infection that most commonly presents with painless haematuria. The condition is diagnosed by identifying schistosomal eggs within the patient's urine and can be treated effectively with oral praziquantel. Untreated, it can cause significant scarring and fibrosis of the urinary tract and may ultimately result in bladder cancer.

4. **Balanitis xerotica obliterans (BXO; also known as lichen sclerosus)**
   BXO is a white, fibrotic lesion affecting the skin of the prepuce that causes phimosis. It also affects the glans penis in about 10% of sufferers and the anterior urethra in about 1%. It can affect boys and adults of all ages and may require circumcision, which is usually curative for preputial BXO. Strong topical steroids are often helpful, especially for diseases affecting the glans penis. It is a lesion that increases the risk of the man subsequently developing penile cancer.

5. **Priapism**
   Priapism is a prolonged erection (greater than 4 hours) that usually arises secondary to sludging of red blood cells within the penis, with progressive ischaemia and damage to the penis. The erection is painful and if left untreated within 12–24 hours will result in complete persistent loss of erectile function. Therefore, such cases need emergency referral to urology. A small proportion (less than 5%) are due to trauma and are paradoxically painless and less urgent. Such a differential is impossible in primary care – so all need urgent referral.

Easily Confused

1. Testicular torsion and epididymitis

Testicular torsion	Epididymitis
Sudden onset testicular pain	Onset of testicular pain, usually gradual
Typically affects children, adolescents and young men	It can affect any age, although rare in children; usually caused by an STI in young men and by a UTI in older men
Testis lies higher, the scrotal skin is often erythematous, the spermatic cord is thickened and the whole hemi-scrotum is exquisitely tender	The scrotal skin is often erythematous and oedematous, the epididymis is thickened and tender and there may be a fever; in severe cases the whole hemi-scrotum is exquisitely tender
Urinalysis is negative	Urinalysis often shows pyuria
Ultrasound will usually show no testicular blood flow	Ultrasound will show hyperaemia of epididymis and possibly testis, with abscess formation sometimes seen

Note: Differentiating between the two is difficult. If there is any doubt, urgent referral is required because the only truly diagnostic test is surgical exploration – and testes that have torted for more than 6 hours are at risk of ischaemic necrosis

2. Overactive bladder and painful bladder syndrome

Overactive bladder	Painful bladder syndrome
Usual symptoms are frequency, urgency, nocturia and, commonly, urge incontinence	Usual symptoms are frequency, urgency and nocturia; incontinence rarely a feature
Pain is not a feature	Pain is a central component of this problem, with pain most prominent when the bladder is full; many women also suffer from dyspareunia
Urgency comprises a painless strong desire to void	Urgency is associated with a strong painful need to pass urine
Stix testing of the urine typically shows no abnormality	Stix testing of the urine is usually positive for leucocytes, and often positive for blood
If this condition is suspected, anticholinergics such as oxybutynin and beta-3 agonists such as mirabegron are the most appropriate first-line therapy	If this condition is suspected, referral for urological assessment and cystoscopy is appropriate

3. Cystitis in males and acute prostatitis

Cystitis in males	Acute prostatitis
Typical symptoms of cystitis, e.g. urgency, frequency and dysuria, possibly with visible haematuria	Typical symptoms of cystitis
Rarely difficulty passing urine	Difficulty passing urine is common
No fever	Fever
Requires a 1-week course of antibiotics	Requires a 1-month course of antibiotics (e.g. ciprofloxacin)
Not unwell enough to warrant admission	May be unwell enough to warrant admission

Prescribing Points

1. **Nitrates and PDE5 inhibitors**
   Patients using PDE5 inhibitors such as sildenafil (Viagra™) or tadalafil (Cialis™) should not use nitrate medication such as GTN because of the risk of significant postural hypotension. This contraindication also applies to nicorandil and the recreational drugs 'poppers', which are also nitric oxide donors and can cause the same side effects.

2. **5-alpha reductase inhibitors and PSA results**
   Drugs such as finasteride or dutasteride, commonly used for the treatment of male LUTS due to benign prostatic hyperplasia, have the effect of reducing PSA levels by around 50%. This is important in the follow-up of men with a raised PSA, in whom a rough adjustment of doubling the measured PSA will give the true PSA level. Alpha-blockers, which are also used in this condition, do not have this effect on PSA.

3. **Drug-related sexual dysfunction**
   A wide range of drugs can cause various sorts of sexual dysfunction as detailed in the following table.

Drug type	Drug or class of drug	Effect
Antihypertensive drugs	Diuretics	Erectile dysfunction (ED)
	Beta blockers	ED
	Centrally acting antihypertensive agents, e.g. clonidine, methyl DOPA	ED
Centrally acting agents	Phenothiazines	ED, reduced libido, ejaculatory dysfunction
	Butyrophenones	ED
	Serotonin reuptake inhibitors	ED, ejaculatory dysfunction
	Tricyclic antidepressants	ED, reduced libido
	Phenytoin	ED, reduced libido
Endocrine drugs	LHRH analogues	ED, reduced libido
	Antiandrogens	ED, reduced libido
	Oestrogens	ED, reduced libido
Recreational drugs	Alcohol	ED, reduced libido, ejaculatory dysfunction
	Marijuana	ED
	Cocaine	ED
	Opiates	ED, reduced libido
	Amphetamines	Reduced libido, ejaculatory dysfunction
	Anabolic steroids	ED, reduced libido
Other drugs	Cimetidine	ED, reduced libido
	Metoclopramide	ED, reduced libido
	Digoxin	ED

4. **Antihypertensives and erectile function**

   While hypertension is a common cause of erectile dysfunction and most antihypertensives make erectile dysfunction worse, the angiotensin-receptor blockers actually improve erectile function. They are therefore the best class of drugs to use in men with hypertension who have co-existent erectile dysfunction.

5. **Antibiotics and urinary tract infections**

   Due to the changing flora that cause urinary tract infections, and due to the varying prevalence of antibiotic resistance, the preferred antibiotic for a urinary infection in a given locality changes with time. It is important to keep up to date with prescribing guidelines for patients with urinary infections, with guidance usually available on local websites.

WOMEN'S HEALTH

Toni Hazell

Ten Pearls of Wisdom

1. You can diagnose osteoporosis without a DEXA scan

There are certain patients whose bone risk is so high that we can assume osteoporosis and treat without a DEXA scan. This might be particularly useful when the wait for a scan is long, preventing your patient from sustaining another fracture in the interim. NICE says that we can consider starting osteoporosis management without a DEXA scan for those with a vertebral fracture. The same might apply to someone whose FRAX score is high enough for a recommendation of treatment without a scan – this would put them in the red zone on the FRAX graphic.

2. The menopause is usually a clinical diagnosis

Women who have symptoms of the menopause and are aged over 45 do not usually need a blood test to diagnose it. Follicle-stimulating hormone (FSH) is raised in the menopause, but it is unreliable in the perimenopause and can sometimes be normal in a menopausal woman. An FSH test may be useful in women who have symptoms of the menopause under the age of 45, although not essential if the diagnosis is clear clinically. Reasons for doing bloods might be to confirm the diagnosis if there is concern about other differentials (e.g. lymphoma as a differential for night sweats), or because you are concerned about premature ovarian insufficiency in a woman under age 40.

3. It's an urban myth that sterilisation is the most effective form of contraception

Given perfect use, oral contraceptives have a 0.3% failure rate – only 3 women per 1,000 will get pregnant each year. In real life, the failure rate is 9%, so of

DOI: 10.1201/9781003304586-32

that same 1,000 women, 90 will face an unwanted pregnancy. Long-acting reversible contraception (LARC) methods do not require regular user input and so their real-life failure rates are the same as that for perfect use. The most effective contraception that we have is the implant, with a failure rate of 0.05%, or 1 pregnancy per year for every 2,000 women who use it. This contrasts favourably with the 0.5% failure rate for sterilisation and also has the benefit of being reversible.

4. Many women with heavy menstrual bleeding (HMB) don't need a pelvic examination or an ultrasound scan

All women with HMB need a full blood count – no other aspect of the examination or investigation is compulsory. If there is no intermenstrual bleeding, pelvic pain or pressure symptoms, consider pharmacological treatment without a physical examination. For most women who need investigation, NICE advises hysteroscopy as the method of choice, with ultrasound being reserved for those women who decline hysteroscopy.

5. The levonorgestrel intrauterine device (LNG-IUD) is a great contraceptive method for women in their 40s

Most women will still need contraception during the perimenopause. The LNG-IUD can do the double job of providing reliable contraception and also acting as the progestogenic component of HRT. Recent FSRH guidance allows for the use of any 52mg LNG-IUD as part of HRT, even though the use of any brand other than Mirena is unlicensed. Remember that use as part of HRT is only for five years, compared to six years for contraception alone.

6. Most cases of chlamydia in women are asymptomatic, but they can still cause damage to fertility

Seventy percent of women with chlamydia have no symptoms. All sexually active people under age 25 are entitled to annual screening, or more frequently if they change partners, via the National Chlamydia Screening Programme. Prolonged exposure to chlamydia due to a lack of treatment or frequent re-infection is a major contributing factor for damage to the fallopian tubes and subsequent subfertility. The prevalence of chlamydia is highest in those under 25, so always advise women in that age group to use a condom as well as reliable contraception.

7. Women with HIV need annual smear tests, even if they have always been normal

Women with HIV are three times more likely to be diagnosed with cervical cancer than women without HIV. Risk factors include a low CD4 count, high viral load and known infection with human papillomavirus (HPV). All women with HIV should have a colposcopy performed at diagnosis, if resources permit, and then annual smears. They can stop having smears at the usual age (currently 65), and they only need to continue if recent smears have been abnormal, following the same protocol as women without HIV. Many smear laboratories have a box to tick on the request form for HIV, which will change the review period to 1 year.

8. Women who are at moderate or high risk of breast cancer may benefit from prophylactic tamoxifen

For women at moderate or high risk of breast cancer, a 5-year course of tamoxifen can reduce the risk of developing breast cancer by 40%, a reduction which persists for at least 16 years after the drug is stopped. Other drugs such as anastrozole and raloxifene have also been used. The NICE guidance on familial breast cancer gives a user-friendly summary of who should be referred for assessment. Local pathways may vary, with the first referral going to either the genetics clinic or the family history breast clinic. Remind women to consider their father's relatives, as it is a common but incorrect myth that only maternal cancers 'count' towards overall risk.

9. Premenstrual syndrome can usually be managed in primary care, but some women will need referral

Premenstrual syndrome (PMS) is defined as 'psychological, physical, and behavioural symptoms occurring in the luteal phase of the normal menstrual cycle'. The severity can vary from mild and transient, to the more severe form, premenstrual dysphoric disorder (PMDD), which can severely affect daily functioning. It is a clinical diagnosis based on the timing of symptoms relative to the menstrual cycle and the only necessary investigations are to exclude any differential diagnoses that are being considered. Management in primary care may include lifestyle changes (diet, exercise, smoking and alcohol reduction), analgesia, hormonal management of the menstrual cycle (e.g. with a combined hormonal contraceptive), and use of an SSRI antidepressant or cognitive behavioural therapy. Referral might result in other treatments such as gonadotrophin-releasing hormone agonists, danazol or surgery.

10. Think about a coagulopathy if heavy periods have occurred since the menarche

Fifty percent of women with HMB have no identifiable cause. For the other half of women, many will have a uterine cause such as fibroids, polyps or malignancy, but a few will have a systemic issue such as the coagulation disorder von Willebrand disease (vWD). If a woman has had HMB since the menarche and has a personal or family history suggesting a coagulation disorder, consider vWD, and check coagulation and von Willebrands factor.

Obscure or Overlooked Diagnoses

1. Bicornuate uterus

A bicornuate uterus results from incomplete fusion of the Müllerian and paramesonephric ducts during embryonic development. There can be several degrees of this, ranging from a uterus with an indentation at the top, all the way through to uterus didelphys where there are two vaginas, two cervices and two single-horned uteri. Women with a bicornuate uterus can usually conceive but may be more likely to have late miscarriages, malpresentations or premature deliveries. The diagnosis may be made on ultrasound or hysteroscopy and can also present with an IUCD failure if the IUCD is in one horn of the uterus and the pregnancy is in the other.

2. Pyometra

A pyometra is a collection of pus which distends the uterine cavity. It is a rare condition, most commonly seen in postmenopausal women or in association with a gynaecological malignancy which has been treated with radiotherapy. Pyometra presents in a similar way to pelvic inflammatory disease, with lower abdominal pain, purulent discharge and fever. On examination, there may be symmetrical uterine enlargement or an acute abdomen due to uterine rupture. Management is surgical, either with a hysterectomy or drainage of the collection.

3. Heterotopic pregnancy

In a heterotopic pregnancy, there is more than one embryo: usually one in the uterine cavity and one in the fallopian tube. This is a rare event, occurring in about 1 in 30,000 of all pregnancies but is more common in those who have used assisted reproduction where it can occur in as many as 1 in 500 pregnancies. When we see a woman with abdominal pain in early pregnancy, ectopic is the key thing to rule out and we are usually reassured by a scan showing an intra-uterine pregnancy. It's important to remember that in rare cases there may be another embryo elsewhere; consider this particularly for women in whom the pain persists/worsens or they become systemically unwell. Heterotopic pregnancies are usually diagnosed in the first trimester, but there has been a case report of a diagnosis as late as 26 weeks gestation.

Easily Confused

1. Urinary tract infection/cystitis and sexually transmitted infection

	Urinary tract infection/cystitis	Sexually transmitted infection
Symptoms in common	Dysuria	Dysuria
Other symptoms	Urinary frequency and urgency Cloudy or smelly urine Nocturia	Increased vaginal discharge Abnormal vaginal bleeding, e.g. after intercourse/between periods Deep dyspareunia
Investigation	None needed in a woman with no haematuria, who is not pregnant or catheterised – treat empirically based on symptoms; otherwise consider urine dipstick and/or send for culture	Swab for chlamydia and gonorrhoea Complete sexual health screen with blood tests for HIV and syphilis Treat empirically before results back if the patient is a contact of a confirmed STI
Management	May depend on locally known sensitivity patterns – in the absence of these, consider nitrofurantoin or trimethoprim first-line	Depends on the suspected STI First-line management of chlamydia is doxycycline or if contraindicated or not tolerated then azithromycin
Possible complications	Ascending infection leading to pyelonephritis, renal abscess, renal failure or sepsis	Ascending infection leading to pelvic inflammatory disease with the risk of sepsis and future tubal infertility, ectopic pregnancy and chronic pelvic pain

2. Secondary dysmenorrhoea and primary dysmenorrhoea

	Secondary dysmenorrhoea	Primary dysmenorrhoea
Cause	Caused by underlying pathology, such as endometriosis, fibroids, pelvic inflammatory disease (PID) or use of an intra-uterine contraceptive device	No identifiable cause – thought to be caused by the production of uterine prostaglandins due to menstruation
Associated symptoms	Subfertility, dyspareunia, menorrhagia, intermenstrual or postcoital bleeding Cyclical bleeding from other sites (e.g. rectal bleeding, nosebleeds) suggests endometriosis	Periods may be associated with nausea, vomiting, fatigue and lower back pain
When did the problem start?	Often after years of painless periods Pain may persist after menstruation finishes, or be present to a lesser degree throughout the cycle but worse during menstruation	Usually starts within 6–12 months of the menarche Pain starts just before menstruation and lasts for up to 3 days
Examination findings	Enlarged uterus from fibroids, adnexal mass from endometrial ovarian cyst, pain from PID A normal examination does not rule out an underlying cause	Usually nothing to find on examination
Management	Treatment of the underlying cause – for women with suspected endometriosis, laparoscopy is needed for diagnosis; some may prefer empirical treatment which avoids surgical intervention	NSAIDs, paracetamol, hormonal contraception or an IUS

Prescribing Points

1. **Women with a uterus always need combined HRT**

   A 52mg LNG-IUD can be used for 5 years for the progestogenic component – if using this, consider writing the date of LNG-IUD change on the prescription for oestrogen.

2. **Extended pill taking**

   There is no need to have a regular break between packets of the combined hormonal contraceptive pill. The FSRH supports extended pill taking, where the pill is taken without a break until there is a breakthrough bleed, at which point the woman has a 4-day break and then restarts. This use of the pill is unlicensed. It can be particularly beneficial in women who have symptoms mainly during their pill-free interval, such as cyclical migraine or pelvic pain.

3. **Emergency contraception**

   Ulipristal is a more effective form of oral emergency contraception than levonorgestrel, but the use of any hormonal contraception in the 5 days after taking ulipristal increases the chance that the ulipristal will fail. Long-term hormonal contraception should therefore not be started in that 5-day window. A copper IUCD is more effective as emergency contraception than either oral method.

4. **High BMI and emergency contraception**

   An increased body mass index (BMI) can reduce the effectiveness of oral emergency contraception. If a woman who weighs more than 70 kg or has a BMI of over 26 kg/m^2 uses levonorgestrel as emergency contraception, she should double the dose to 3 mg. In most cases, a copper IUCD or ulipristal will be more suitable.

5. **Transdermal hormone replacement therapy**

   Transdermal hormone replacement therapy carries no increased risk of venous thromboembolism (VTE) compared to the baseline population risk, and should therefore be first-line for women at increased risk of VTE, including those with a BMI of over 30 kg/m^2.

6. **Bleeding with contraceptive implant**

   The mechanism of troublesome bleeding with the contraceptive implant is poorly understood and management can be difficult. Treatment options include a trial of the combined pill as well as the implant (unlicensed), or a short course of mefenamic acid. There is inadequate evidence to recommend the use of the progesterone-only pill to control implant-related bleeding, though it is sometimes used. Other suggestions to control such bleeding have included doxycycline, tamoxifen, ulipristal or misoprostol, but these are not recommended either due to lack of evidence of benefit or lack of evidence for no effect on the contraceptive efficacy of the implant.

7. **Resources**

The BNF is often not helpful for prescribing in women who are pregnant or breastfeeding. Better resources include BUMPS (best use of medicines in pregnancy; www.medicinesinpregnancy.org/Medicine--pregnancy/), UKTIS (UK Teratology Information Service; www.uktis.org), the Breastfeeding Network (www.breastfeedingnetwork.org.uk) and the Specialist Pharmacy Service (www.sps.nhs.uk/home/guidance/safety-in-breastfeeding/). Some of these sites have downloadable information leaflets aimed at patients.

8. **Women with depression during pregnancy or postnatally**

Women with depression during pregnancy or in the postnatal period can usually safely take antidepressants. Ideally, they should all be under the care of a specialist perinatal mental health team. Never stop antidepressants abruptly. Urgent referral is indicated for severe depression, self-neglect and pregnancy in a woman with a history of known severe mental illness such as bipolar disorder or puerperal psychosis.

9. **Starting contraception**

All contraceptive methods can be started at any time in the cycle if you are 'reasonably certain' that the woman is not pregnant – see the FSRH guidance for the definition of reasonably certain. If you cannot be reasonably certain, then you can still quick-start most methods (including the copper IUCD if the criteria for emergency contraception are met), but not the LNG-IUD. The depot injection is less suitable in this situation. Women who start contraception where there is uncertainty about pregnancy must do a pregnancy test 21 days after the last episode of unprotected intercourse.

INDEX

W

X

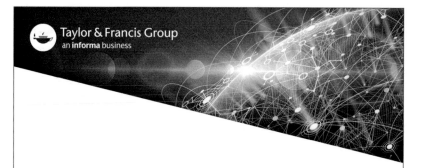